CHIROPRACTIC FIRST

The Fastest Growing Healthcare Choice... Before Drugs or Surgery

Terry A. Rondberg, D.C.

WHAT READERS ARE SAYING

"Humanity desperately needs a solution to the health care crisis—Chiropractic First provides that answer in a clear and uncompromising way. Every D.C. should make this book a 'must read' for new patients."

— Christopher Kent, DC
President of the Council on Chiropractic Practice (CCP)

"Extremely educational and thoroughly enjoyable... Dr. Rondberg writes in a clear, concise style that is easy to follow and hold the reader's attention. He takes the reader through a step-by-step account of how the body works, what chiropractic is, and how chiropractic can enhance our health and wellness."

— Pamela Hertzberg
Chiropractic Assistant (CA)

"...bringing a new, clear dynamic insight to Chiropractors, patients and the public, your book is on my must-read list. Everyone better read this book now!"

— Guy Riekeman, D.C.
President, Palmer Chiropractic University

CHIROPRACTIC FIRST

The Fastest Growing Healthcare Choice...
Before Drugs or Surgery

Published by Dr. Terry A. Rondberg, DC

Copyright 1996, 1998, 2015
First Printing by Chiropractic Journal 1996 –
Second Printing by Chiropractic Journal 1998 –
    ISBN: 0-9647168-2-8
Third Printing by Dr. Terry A. Rondberg (CreateSpace)
Paperback, 2015
    ISBN–13: 978-1514146965
    ISBN–10: 1514146967

First Kindle Edition – June, 2015

Library of Congress Catalog Number: 95-92554
ISBN: 0-9647168-2-8

Photographs of Daniel D. Palmer and Bartlett J. Palmer with permission from the Palmer College of Chiropractic.

*I dedicate this book
to my mother, Lois Lee Rondberg,
for introducing me to chiropractic,
to my father, Daniel Rondberg, who
always supported me in my ideals,
and
to my daughters,
Brooke and Shannon.
Thank you for all your love
and understanding.*

CONTENTS

Chiropractic first, drugs second and surgery last...

CHIROPRACTIC
By B.J. Palmer

We chiropractors work with the subtle substance of the soul. We release the prisoned impulses, a tiny rivulet of force that emanates from the mind and flows over the nerves to the cells and stirs them to life. We deal with the magic power that transforms common food into living, loving, thinking clay; that robes the earth with beauty, and hues and scents the flowers with the glory of the air.

In the dim, dark distant long ago, when the sun first bowed to the morning star, this power spoke and there was life, it quickened the slime of the sea and the dust of the earth and drove the cell to union with its fellows in countless living forms. Through eons of time it finned the fish and winged the bird and fanged the beast. Endlessly it worked, evolving its forms until it produced the crowning glory of them all. With tireless energy it blows the bubble of each individual life and then silently, relentlessly dissolves the form and absorbs the spirit into itself again.

And yet you asked, "Can chiropractic cure appendicitis or the flu?" Have you more faith in a knife or a spoonful of medicine than in the power that animates the living world?

Chapter 1
Adjusting to a Better Life

I had only been in practice about a year when I first met Mrs. Hoffman. She was recently divorced and working as a waitress to support her children. During our initial consultation, she complained of back pain and said that her back started hurting when she was lifting heavy trays of food. I explained that I adjusted the spine to help the overall body operate at its peak efficiency not directly to alleviate back pain but to correct any nerve interference I found. I told her that often, when I make an adjustment, the patient's back pain disappears. It didn't matter what symptom or condition a person had, he or she would benefit from the correction of nerve interference, resulting in improved nerve supply.

Mrs. Hoffman also asked if I thought I could help her son, Richie, who was "in really bad shape." I said I could usually help "if the patient is alive and has a nervous system." Hope was reflected in her eyes.

Richie was one of seven-year-old twin boys. His brother, Johnny, was just fine, healthy and active. Richie, however, was a different story. He was dying. He had been seen by seventeen different doctors and not one of them could agree on a diagnosis. In seven years, over thirty-seven different medications had been prescribed for him. He was in the hospital twice for tests and observation. Each time, his stay had been extended and the family's insurance had paid tens of thousands of dollars for Richie's medical expenses. (Now, the family had no insurance because Mr. Hoffman had stopped paying the premiums after the divorce.)

The last time he was hospitalized, the baffled doctors felt Richie's condition was hopeless and sent him home with instructions that his mother should make him as comfortable as possible until his death. Currently, Richie was taking five different medications, including the drug Phenobarbital, which is used to control seizures.

Mrs. Hoffman received this dire verdict about a week before she came to see me for back pain.

After listening to her story, I told her I would examine Richie for nerve interference, and she was not to worry about payment. I referred to the sign in our waiting room which said: "We accept all patients regardless of their condition or financial ability to pay."

When I saw a Richie, I must admit I was quite shocked by his physical condition. Mrs. Hoffman had to carry him in her arms into my office. Because of his condition, he had never been able to wear shoes and was dressed only in shorts and a T-shirt. He seemed to have no body or facial hair and his frail body was covered with sores from head to toe.

On his legs, the sores were so profuse that I couldn't see any healthy skin. Furthermore he was so drugged from the five different medications he was taking that his eyes were rolling back in his head. Richie really looked closer to death than anyone I have ever seen. His brother Johnny had come with them and the contrast between the two children made Richie's situation all the more dramatic.

It was difficult to examine the boy. I was so moved by his condition, I actually had to leave the examining room to regain my composure. When I returned and examined him, I explained to his mother that Richie had nerve interference in his neck. I told her I would adjust him every day for a while. Even though it was illegal for me to give advice about medications, I went so far as to tell her that if Richie were my child, I would slowly try to reduce his medications.

We agreed that I would adjust Mrs. Hoffman and both her sons for five dollars a week. I had found nerve interference in Johnny's spine even though he said he felt great. I wanted to adjust him before he developed symptoms.

After I'd been working with the family for about six weeks, I began to get discouraged. I didn't see any real change in Richie's condition and I wondered if his mother noticed this too, and felt disappointed.

When I questioned her as to whether or not she thought the adjustments were helping him, I have never forgotten what she said to me. I was a young doctor then, but many years later, I still carry her message of faith with me. Mrs. Hoffman said:

"When I first came to you, I also suffered with severe headaches and menstrual cramps I never told you about. I was taking a lot of medication which I now no longer need. I feel great except for my back, but it seems improved.

"You explained how the power that made my body is the only power that could heal it and I knew you were talking about God. I understand that it may be too late for Richie because he has been sick so long, but, if you give up on him, I have no other place to go for help.

"Your adjustments have already helped me so much, I just know that if it's God's will for Richie to recover, then he is going to get better. Please don't give up, Dr. Rondberg."

How could I do anything but agree to continue the adjustments? I cast aside my own discouragement and lack of faith, and made a promise to myself that I would never again doubt the ability of my adjustments or the hope they offered.

The very next week, the miracle began to unfold. Richie's mother excitedly showed me some areas of clear skin, where earlier there had only been open bloody sores. (She had gradually reduced his medication.)

The child continued to make progress, and at the end of eight weeks of care, it was obvious that his body was healing at an amazing rate. He was excited about the hair fuzz growing on top of his head. Furthermore, he was walking into my office now, and he was proudly wearing his first pair of shoes.

It took several more months for Richie to be completely healed. Finally, the only reminders of his condition or areas of skin that were marked with the pinkish coloration where the open sores had been.

I never found out the correct name for Richie's medical condition because none of the experts could agree on a diagnosis. The only thing Mrs. Hoffman and I cared about was that Richie got his life back. It was stunning proof that with an improved spinal structure, the potential for a healthy body and normal function can return.

And I will always be grateful for the lesson I learned about not giving up on any patient regardless of his or her disease. I have always limited my practice objective to specific adjusting for the correction of nerve interference. I give each of my patients the opportunity to receive care that helps eliminate the interference to their body's natural expression of Innate Wisdom.

OPTIMAL HEALTH CARE

If you could create the most satisfying healing system imaginable, what would you recommend?

Most of us would want a natural method; one that utilizes the body's own abilities to promote internal healing and ongoing wellness. Dangerous drugs would not be used and frightening surgeries would not be performed.

If it sounds like such a system is too good to be true, you are in for a pleasant surprise. There is such a system of healing. While the roots of manipulation are in antiquity, true chiropractic began in 1895. To date, millions of people have benefited from this non-medical—and drug free healthcare.

Chiropractic is the largest natural primary healthcare profession in the world. It's one of the most praised, yet most misunderstood of all the healthcare disciplines, despite the fact that more than 25 million Americans utilize it each year. It's practiced by 50,000 doctors around the world and is licensed in every state in the union. In accredited colleges in America, Japan, England, Australia, Canada, France and South Africa more than 7500 students are studying this discipline.

HISTORY OF CHIROPRACTIC

If you think that chiropractic is a new science, it is. However, you will be surprised to know the first pictures depicting spinal manipulation were discovered in prehistoric cave paintings in Point le Merd, in southwestern France. They may have been crude, nonspecific attempts to manipulate the spine, but these early historical records date back to 17,500 B.C. The ancient Chinese were using manipulation in 2700 B.C.; Greek papyruses, from 1500 B.C., gave directions for solving low back problems by maneuvering the legs. We also know that the ancient Japanese, Egyptians, Babylonians, Hindus, Tibetans and Syrians all practiced spinal manipulation. Even in Tahiti, there is evidence that manipulative therapy has been used for centuries.

Historical records in Egypt reveal that men and women were stronger and healthier when their backs were straight instead of twisted. The Egyptians were very concerned with correcting the spine.

Ancient American Indian hieroglyphics showed *back walking* (that is, walking on the back of a patient) being practiced as a method of curing the sick. The Sioux, Winnebago and Creek Indians in North America all left records of manipulation and healing. In Mexico and Central America, the Mayan, Aztec, call Toltec, Tarascan, and Zoltec Indians routinely used manipulation. American Incas were sophisticated enough to develop manipulation into a well-defined and well-documented art.

Hippocrates was a Greek physician who died in 377 BC. He wrote over seventy books on healing and was a proponent of spinal manipulation. He believed that only nature could heal and it was the physician's duty to remove any obstruction that would prevent the body from healing.

"Get knowledge of the spine, for this is the requisite for many diseases."
— Hippocrates, 460-377 B.C.

Hippocrates believed that the essence of life and the natural healing ability of the body were the result of a *vital spirit*. That same concept of "vitalism" occurred throughout ancient writings. In the 20th century, vitalism was replaced by the idea of an Innate Intelligence.

Herodotus, a contemporary of Hippocrates, gained fame curing diseases by correcting spinal abnormalities through therapeutic exercises. If the patient was too weak to exercise, Herodotus would manipulate the patient's spine. The philosopher Aristotle was critical of Herodotus' tonic-free approach because, "...he made old men young and thus prolonged their lives too greatly." This would be considered a benefit today, but it was disconcerting in early Greece where the life expectancy was very limited— not more than three decades.

In Greece, crude mechanical devices were invented to stretch the spine and correct dislocations. Archaeologists have also uncovered pictures of Greek patients being hung upside down by their heels. Physicians also walked on patient's backs to correct spinal deviations.

In Rome, by the Second Century A.D., Claudius Galen taught the proper positions and relations of the vertebrae and the spinal column. Galen was known as the *Prince of Physicians*, a title he was given after he aligned the neck vertebrae of a well-known Roman scholar whose right hand was paralyzed. Once the vertebra was aligned, nerve transmission was restored and the scholar was able to use his hand again. Galen's reputation was made!

The skills of spinal manipulation were handed down within families, and almost every village posted a "bone-setter" who could cure by straightening the spine. In both Eastern and Western cultures manipulation of soft tissues or massage were recognized as a useful component in healthcare.

Crude types of manipulation continued all over the world until Daniel David (D.D.) Palmer discovered the correct specific spinal adjustment. It was his son, B.J. Palmer, who later developed it into the modern philosophy, art and science of chiropractic we are familiar with today.

D.D. Palmer thought that commonly used drugs and potions were actually toxic and created stress for ill patients. He was more interested in finding the cause of the disease and eliminating it through natural means.

"I am not the first person to replace subluxated vertebrae, but I do plan to be the first person to replace displaced vertebrae by using the spinous and transverse processes as levers… and to develop the philosophy and science of chiropractic adjustments."
—D.D. Palmer, Discoverer of Chiropractic

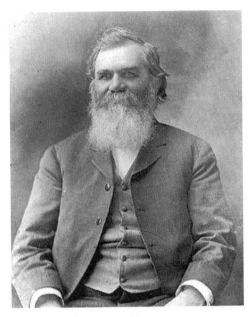

D. D. Palmer was born in Ontario, Canada, in 1845. He moved to the United States when he was 20 years old. He spent the years after the Civil War teaching school, raising bees, and selling sweet raspberries in the Iowa and Illinois river towns along the bluffs on either side of the Mississippi River. While living in What Cheer, Iowa in 1885, D. D. became familiar with the work of Paul Caster, a magnetic healer who had some success in Ottumwa. He then moved his family to Burlington, near Ottumwa, to learn the techniques of magnetic healing. This was a common therapy.

At the time, practitioners used the body's natural

magnetic properties for healing purposes. Two years later, he moved his family again, this time to Davenport, Iowa, where he opened the Palmer Cure and infirmary.

On September 18, 1895, D.D. Palmer performed his first adjustment on a janitor, Harvey Lillard, who had been deaf for seventeen years. The man's hearing returned, and because of the success of Palmer's spinal adjustment, the modern recorded history of chiropractic began.

Here is the description of this event in D.D. Palmer's own words:

"Harvey Lillard... could not hear the racket of a wagon on the street or the ticking of a watch. I made inquiry as to the cause of his deafness and was informed that when he was exerting himself in a cramped, stooping position, he felt something give way in his back and immediately became deaf.

"An examination showed a vertebra rack from its normal position. I reasoned that if the vertebra was replaced, the man's hearing should be restored. With this object in view, a half hour's talk persuaded Mr. Lillard to allow me to replace it. I racked it into position by using the spinous process as a lever, and soon the man could hear as before.

"There was nothing accidental about this as it was accomplished with an object in view, and the result expected was

*obtained. There was nothing 'crude' about this adjust-
ment; it was specific, so much so that no other Chiropractor has equaled it."*

Over the succeeding months, other patients came to
him with diverse problems including flu, sciatica, migraine
headaches, stomach complaints, and epilepsy and heart
problems. D.D. Palmer found each of these conditions responded well to the adjustments which he was calling
"hand treatments." Later he coined the term chiropractic,
from the Greek words, *chiro*, meaning (hand) and *practic*,
meaning (practice or operation). He renamed his clinic
the Palmer School & Infirmary of Chiropractic.

The term "Infirmary" (implying medicinal treatment)
was confusing because none of the patients were given
medicines of any kind. They hadn't undergone surgery.
Under Palmer's care fevers broke, pain ended, infections
healed, vision improved, stomach disorders disappeared,
and of course, hearing returned. Palmer knew what to do
for these people. What he didn't know was *why* his treatments were so effective.

Often surprised at the effectiveness of his adjustments, D.D. Palmer returned to his studies of anatomy
and physiology to learn more about the vital connection
between the spine and one's health. He realized spinal
adjustments were correcting vertebral subluxations,
(nerve interference), that was causing the patients' complaints. Based on the body's Innate ability to heal itself,
and aided by the practitioner's ability to correct the nerve

interference—chiropractic often brings an end to needless suffering from pain and discomfort in natural ways unknown in any other health discipline. It is one of the most powerful and effective healing methods available today.

Yet at first, even though it proved to be a successful way of healing the body, chiropractic adjustments were not readily accepted.

Years after Harvey Lillard's hearing was restored, the news media delighted in vilifying the pioneer chiropractor. D.D. Palmer was labeled a "charlatan" and a "crank on magnetism." The medical community, afraid of his success and discouraged by its own failure to heal diseases, joined the crusade and wrote letters to the editors of local papers, openly criticizing his methods and accusing him of practicing medicine without a license.

D.D. Palmer defended himself against the doctors attacked by presenting arguments against the medical procedures of vaccination and surgery. He also cautioned against introducing medicine into the body saying it was often unnecessary and even harmful.

In 1905, the medical establishment won a minor victory when they conspired to have D.D. Palmer indicted for practicing medicine without a license. He was sentenced to 105 days in jail and was required to pay a $350 dollar fine.

At first, he argued with the judge and refused to pay the fine. (The local newspapers gave a lot of coverage to this incident.) After serving twenty-three days of his sentence, however, he paid the fine and was released.

From 1906 to 1913, D.D. Palmer published two books, *The Science of Chiropractic* and *The Chiropractor's Adjuster*. He died in Los Angeles at the age of sixty-eight, after after being stricken by typhoid fever.

The world owes much to D.D. Palmer. His son B.J. once stated that he felt his father D.D. had done more for mankind than any other single individual and should be compared with other great men such as Thomas Edison.

"I desired to know why one person was ailing and his associate, eating at the same table, working in the same shop... was not. Why? What difference was there in the two persons that caused one to have [disease] while his partner... escaped? Why?
— D.D. Palmer, Discoverer of Chiropractic

B.J. PALMER

It was D.D. Palmer's son, Bartlett Joshua Palmer, who is credited with *developing* chiropractic. Born in 1881, B.J., as he was always called, was a prolific author and speaker who was in great demand by audiences worldwide. He had an extraordinary gift as a salesman and his product was chiropractic.

By all accounts, B.J. was as much of a character as his father. He loved to tell stories which were more than a little embellished to make them more entertaining and he thoroughly enjoyed talking to the people who eagerly gathered around him.

Even though B.J. had seen very little of his father when he was growing up, when they did get together, they discovered they had similar temperaments and often clashed violently.

B. J. Palmer

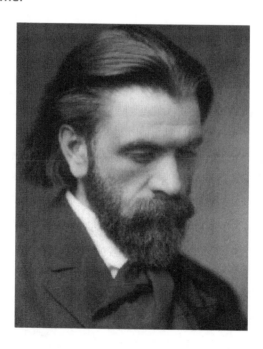

One time after an argument D.D. abruptly packed up and moved from Davenport to Portland, Oregon, where he opened the Pacific College of Chiropractic.

The senior Palmer then went on to Santa Barbara, California, to establish another chiropractic clinic, leaving

B.J. to cope with the struggling school in Iowa.

Like most great men, B.J. is remembered for his many idiosyncrasies, several of which were embarrassing to his family. He was very adamant about going to bed early in the evening so he could rise at five in the morning to spend several hours writing. Promptly at nine, even if guests were present, he would loosen his tie, take off his shoes, carry them upstairs, and announce that the evening was over—at least as far as he was concerned.

When he went to bed, it was imperative his head was pointed toward the North Pole and his feet to the South. This was how he felt he got the most restful sleep, as he felt the earth's currents would flow through him properly. This belief was so strong that even when he traveled, he would rearrange the hotel furniture to accommodate this need, no matter how late the hour or how inconvenient the restructuring of the room.

Before air-conditioning became commonplace, B.J. would go to bed on the screened-in porch wearing a night-shirt he had soaked in cold water. He believed the evaporation of the water cooled him naturally.

On the third floor of B.J.'s home, he and his father kept their renowned collection of human spines. The spinal columns were hung in rows along the walls and provided an invaluable resource for students at the Palmer School of Chiropractic—as well as endless amusement for B.J.'s son, David, and other youngsters in the neighborhood. As a young boy, David was often asked to perform for company by reciting from memory of the 206 bones in the body. This was an accomplishment B.J. felt was more important than playing a musical instrument or memorizing poetry.

B.J. never tasted alcohol, but he did chain-smoke cheap cigars which were manufactured in West Davenport. He only smoked expensive cigars when they were given to him as a gift. While B.J. Palmer was a man of somewhat unorthodox habits, he was the perfect person to carry on his father's work and defend the fledgling profession against its detractors. Because of his efforts, chiropractic survived, and was rightfully acknowledged as bringing relief and maintaining health without first resorting to medications.

B.J. felt a deep concern for his father's clinic and infirmary, and felt responsible for continuing the school from which he himself had graduated in 1902. From the time of his graduation, he became a teacher at the school and also had a private chiropractic practice. In 1905, he moved the school in clinic to a large Victorian home on Brady Street Hill in Davenport, Iowa. The building was partitioned to provide living quarters for B.J. and his young wife, Mabel, who had graduated that same year from the Palmer School. The house also included sleeping quarters for the students and classrooms in the basement.

Through his own efforts, B.J. became a highly educated person who was respected by the civic and financial leaders in Davenport. Under his picture in the gallery of distinguished citizens of Davenport, a plaque reads: "B.J. Palmer, world-renowned as spokesman-developer of his father's discovery of chiropractic. Famed educator, traveler, author, radio-television pioneer (WOC-radio and TV), among the nation's first. President, Palmer College of Chiropractic, 1905-1961."

B.J. Palmer believed that nothing was impossible if you work hard enough. He used to say: "Only the hen can make money by laying around." He developed the chiropractic philosophy, art and science, into a profession at a time when it was little more than a loosely knit structure.

He enabled the Palmer college graduates to be licensed and qualified to practice chiropractic. During the 1920s, the school enrollment was over two thousand students. While other chiropractic schools were springing up all over the world, not one of them was as large as Palmer College.

B.J. Palmer has been described as controversial, visionary, outspoken, eccentric, energetic, single-minded and opinionated. Every one of these terms is appropriate. No one else traveled as much, fought as many court battles, or successfully introduced as much legislation to improve the profession. In 1926, he became president of the International Chiropractors Association; the position he held until his death in 1961. During those years, he fought to have chiropractors licensed by separate licensing boards, all the while carrying on a public feud with Morris Fishbein who was the editor of the *Journal of the American Medical Association*.

In 1910, B.J. advocated the use of Wilhelm Roentgen's invention, the x-ray machine, as a valid tool in the practice of chiropractic. Within the faculty there was a divided philosophy about the use of equipment of any sort. Some of them were so infuriated that they left Palmer College to form their own training facility which they named Universal Chiropractic College. To add fuel to the fire, D.D. Palmer chose to ally himself with the new school, as a slap in the face to his son. D.D. had never forgiven his son for following the advice of his attorney. When D.D. was put in jail four years earlier, the attorney advised that the school's assets be put in his wife's name to protect them. Eventually Universal Chiropractic College closed and was forgotten.

One of B.J.'s strongest weapons in the battle to defend and validate chiropractic was the fledgling medium, commercial radio. By 1922, he and his family had moved away from the school to an imposing residence further up the Brady Street Hill. Inspired by his son David's fascination with ham radio, B.J. bought a 250-watt amateur radio station. Called it WOC (Wonders of Chiropractic) and it became the keystone of the Palmer Communications empire. At first, the station was a family-run affair but it soon became the first 500-watt radio station in the United States. In 1927, it became the westernmost link of the tiny new NBC network. B.J. became so proficient at using the new medium to move people to action, that he wrote a book, *Radio Salesmanship*, which became an essential textbook for anyone in the industry.

After his death, the Davenport times said that B.J.: "...observed that the most effective announcers were those who use as few words as possible to get their point across, and who adopted a positive attitude." Former President Ronald Reagan was employed by B.J. as a radio announcer at WOC.

B.J. loved epigrams and slogans which he collected and shared with others by painting them on walls, stairwells and chimneys all around the campus. He had two sayings that he felt were particularly meaningful: *"The world makes a path for the man who knows where he's going."* and *"Early to bed, early to rise, work like hell and advertise, makes a man healthy, wealthy and wise."*

While many of these sayings were his own, B.J. had a special fondness for the words of Mark Twain, Abraham Lincoln, Zane Grey and Teddy Roosevelt.

Earl Ackerman managed the Blackhawk Hotel in Davenport, and he was a good friend of B.J. Palmer. He wrote: "Like his father, B.J. subscribed wholeheartedly to the idea of inner intelligence, the 'Innate,' as they called it. I don't think you could talk to B.J. within a period of 48 hours, say, when he wouldn't mention the word 'Innate' at least a half-dozen times. It was a part of his teaching. He thought that each of us has the 'Innate' within us and that it controls what we do as well as our health. Still, each of us is responsible for what we do, for living a life of accomplishment, but in a way, this all comes from within ourselves."

Today every doctor of chiropractic owes B.J. Palmer a great debt. Without B.J.'s relentless work over his lifetime, the profession of chiropractic would have ended in 1913, along with the passing of D.D. Palmer, instead of flourishing as we continue it into the 21st century.

"THINK! SPEAK! ACT POSITIVE! I AM! I WILL! I CAN! I MUST!"
—B.J. Palmer, D.C.

MODERN CHIROPRACTIC

THE CHIROPRACTIC PRACTICE OBJECTIVE: The professional practice objective of chiropractic is to correct vertebral subluxations also referred to as nerve interference, in a safe and effective manner. The correction of nerve interference is not considered to be a specific cure for any particular symptom or disease. It is applicable to any patient who exhibits nerve interference regardless of the presence or absence of symptoms or disease.

Today, chiropractic has come a long way from D.D. Palmer's practice in Davenport, Iowa. Specifically, the chiropractor determines the presence of nerve interference and helps the body correct itself by introducing a force in a prescribed manner. Contrary to popular misinformation, the doctor of chiropractic (D.C.) doesn't force the misaligned vertebrae back into place but he or she facilitates the body's correction of nerve interference.

During the adjustment, the subluxated vertebrae are unlocked and released from their misaligned positions. The body's inborn intelligence is called upon to shape the spine. When this happens, the vertebrae return to their proper alignment and the normal nerve supply is restored. This allows one to achieve maximum healing potential with a complete nerve supply.

This book explains what chiropractic is, how it works and what it can do for you and your family. In no way am I suggesting that you should never consult a medical physician. There are surgeries that must be performed, and wounds, broken bones and internal injuries that require medical treatment. However, you will realize that when confronted with a physical problem, your safest and most effective first choice for general healthcare should be a chiropractor. You will understand why medicine should be used as a last resort—when the body cannot heal itself without intervention.

Wisdom dictates that you begin the healing process with conservative care that doesn't cause any side effects.

My recommendation:
Chiropractic first, drugs second and surgery last.

DON'T LET YOUR SPINE GET ON YOUR NERVES

The purpose of chiropractic care is the correction of nerve interference. Nerve interference promotes sickness and disease. It robs our vitality and weakens our immune system.

The spinal column consists of 24 small bones called vertebrae. Seven of these are located in the neck. Twelve are found in the mid-back, and five are in the lower back.

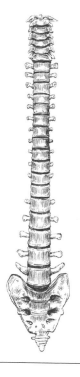
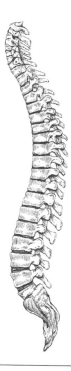

It's very rare to find someone with the spine that's perfectly aligned. In most people, the spine curves slightly to the right or the left, and sometimes, one or more of the vertebrae are twisted or rotated.

When the vertebrae are misaligned, the flow of messages from the brain to all the other cells in the body is distorted. This type of nerve interference creates disorganization of bodily processes and dis-ease. This misalignment of the vertebrae can often exist undetected and slowly undermine health.

DISEASE OR DIS-EASE?

The word *disease*, is a combination of *dis* and *ease*. *Dis* is a prefix meaning "apart from" and *ease* meaning a "state of balance." It follows then that dis-ease is a lack of comfort, a loss of harmony in the system. When there is a lack of harmony in music, the musician adjusts the notes to complement one another and "work well together." That's exactly what an adjustment to correct or reduce nerve interference can do—restore body harmony.

Unlike music, where discord is immediately apparent, damage from nerve interference is not so obvious at first.

The unfortunate aspect of this "dis-ease" is that it need not be painful to silently destroy the body's health and well-being. Gradually, the body's life-support systems begin to fail, and the ability to live a full life diminishes. Nerve interference is often referred to as a ***silent killer***, because it may be present for many years before symptoms arise. It can quietly, painlessly undermine your health before any major warning signs appear.

The causes of nerve interference are numerous and

often, unavoidable. They can be caused at birth if the delivery is difficult or requires the use of forceps. Many births result in subluxations. Children, during the critical growing years, fall while learning to walk. In later years they engage in activities like skateboarding or surfing and many other kinds of sports which can cause subluxations. Other spinal problems can be caused by a junk food diet or having poor sleeping positions. Many seemingly harmless activities can disturb the integrity of the nerve system.

As adults, many things can weaken the spine, and cause nerve interference. This list includes: sports accidents, automobile collisions, and falls in the house, bad posture, and emotional stress, dental problems, pushing ourselves past our limits, alcohol and drug abuse or even carrying heavy briefcases or handbags on a daily basis.

We've reached a point where nerve interference is epidemic in our population. To ignore it and not have your spine checked regularly by a chiropractor, is to invite disease to overwhelm your body and impair the quality of your life. In later chapters, we will be exploring the connection between your spine and various physical conditions we tend to consider an unavoidable part of our human condition. You will understand the vital role your spine plays in your life, and gain new insights on how you can promote and maintain good health, with less fear of needing dangerous chemicals and/or invasive surgery.

"To take in a new idea you must destroy the old, let go of old opinions, to observe and conceive new thoughts. To learn is but to change your opinion."
— B.J. Palmer, D.C.

A doctor of chiropractic is uniquely trained to locate and help correct nerve system interference which promotes the body's natural healing ability.

Chapter 2
Chiropractic 101

To understand chiropractic, one must have a basic understanding about how the body functions. This chapter and the next will explain our marvelous machine, the body.

From the time you were born, your Inner Wisdom has known exactly how to keep you healthy and alive. It knows how fast your heart should beat, how often your lungs need to breathe, how to digest food and how to eliminate waste. There are millions of details controlled by your Inner Wisdom to keep this marvelous machine in prime functioning condition.

"... a kind of kind of super intelligence exists in each of us, infinitely smarter and possessed of technical know-how far beyond our present understanding."
— Lewis Thomas, M.D.

Every living organism in our world possesses what chiropractors call Innate Intelligence. The body machine comes out of the "factory" fully able to function, as long as it has regular fuel and adequate maintenance.

Innate Intelligence sends instructions to every organ and cell in your body through the nervous system housed by the vertebrae. However, unless your spinal vertebrae are correctly aligned, those instructions can't be received and followed properly. The result is "dis-ease" and dysfunction.

THE PHILOSOPHY OF CHIROPRACTIC

While the word *philosophy* may bring to mind ancient Greeks or bearded scholars in dusty libraries, the philosophy of health is a vibrant study that influences how we live. It helps us make critical choices about how we treat our bodies.

Too often, people respond to every symptom by gulping down pills to alleviate the discomfort. When they catch a cold, they buy an over-the-counter remedy from the drugstore. If they gain a few pounds, they head for the diet pills. When they feel tired, they take pills to stay awake and when they want to sleep, there's a pill to take for that too.

There is a bottle of pills to combat headaches and another for irregularity and still another for diarrhea. If you have a symptom, the drug companies have a remedy.

The message to the consumer is, whatever is wrong, just pop a pill and you will be fine. We call this the "Medical Philosophy of Disease."

Every one of us has symptoms from time to time. When something goes wrong in the body, we get a rash, feel pain or experience discomfort in any one of a hundred ways. The body's warning system is at work. Like the red lights on your car's dashboard, symptoms tell you it's time to check something in your internal machinery. For the followers of the medical philosophy of disease, these warnings are treated by attempting to fix the symptoms and not the cause. These people believe something from the outside will change something on the inside. That state of mind is dangerous to one's health.

Let's go back to the car analogy. Say the oil light comes on. What are you going to do? Pull into your nearest gas station and put a quart of oil in the engine or are you going to disconnect the light so you won't see it? The logical answer doesn't require much thought. Back to your body; if you get a pain in your head, are you going to check out the cause and correct it? Or are you going to take a painkiller and assume the problem is gone because the symptom has been alleviated?

"Each patient carries his own doctor inside him. They come to us not knowing that truth. We are at our best when we give the doctor who resides within each patient a chance to work."
— Albert Schweitzer, M.D.

When you realize your body is somewhat similar to a machine, then it's obvious what the answer has to be. You recognize the need to fix the internal mechanism so the machine is working well again. That's the "Philosophy of Health." It's the belief that health comes from within. A properly functioning body can do everything naturally that pills attempt to do chemically. Furthermore, the body knows when to heal, how to heal and when to stop healing and go back on maintenance.

If you cut your hand, what would you do? Of course, you'd clean the cut, applying a topical antibacterial cream and bandage the wound to keep it clean while it's healing. So far, so good. But these are *external* treatments.

What would you suggest your body do *internally*? Would you think to have your tissues swell to cut off the blood flow to the cut? How about sending special chemicals to the area so the blood will clot? Would you remember to send extra white blood cells to prevent infection?

The fact is, if you had to stop and try to remember all these steps, your hand would fall off before you figured out how to heal it. Fortunately, you're Innate Intelligence knows how to heal this kind of wound. It also knows what to do when you get a cold, hurt your back, get a headache or have an allergic reaction.

The purpose of healthcare should be to allow the body's wisdom to do the healing without interfering with this process. When you use chemicals or surgical procedures at the outset, you interfere with your body's intelligence and interfere with the healing functions before you know if your body's wisdom is adequate to correct the problem.

Chiropractic philosophy begins with the premise that there is an order to the universe. Nothing is random or meaningless in our world. There is a reason for everything.

Granted, we may not always recognize that reason, let alone understand it, but we can be certain that nothing occurs by chance or "just happens."

We know that there is an intelligent order to the universe. A guiding force exists in all living matter, and most definitely in human beings. It's only because of this intelligence that we can continue to exist and operate in this world. Without it, our planet would be a shapeless pile of rocks and debris. Plants wouldn't know how to grow. The animals wouldn't know how to breed and replenish their species. Birds wouldn't know how to fly, or fish how to swim.

Now, this premise isn't a matter of blind faith or religious faith on the part of scientists, philosophers and chiropractors. It's based on physical evidence seen in the real world.

Look around you! Can everything in the universe be the result of random selection or luck? Why is a bird's wing perfectly designed for flight, right down to the tiniest pinfeather? Does it just happen that a plants roots travel downward into the ground and its leaves grow upward? If the universe were really random, at least some plants would send the roots straight up and bury their leaves in the soil. The sun would only come up on random days and it would be difficult to be certain of anything occurring again.

To think the universe is operating without any intelligent plan is like thinking that the Great Sphinx of Egypt was the result of an accidental rock slide!

UNIVERSAL INTELLIGENCE

Innate intelligence is within Universal Intelligence which guides all life. Innate Intelligence is in every living thing. It is revealed when a plant turns its leaves toward the light or when a bird sits on its eggs until they hatch and when a human body knows what to do to heal itself.

Concepts like Universal Intelligence and Innate Intelligence greatly influence your health and your life. Once understood, you will see why your body always strives to remain healthy. You'll also learn what your body sometimes needs help to function normally and achieve its goal of optimum health and well-being.

"Intelligence is present everywhere in our bodies... our own inner intelligence is far superior to any we can try to substitute from the outside."
— Deepak Chopra, M.D.

It requires human intelligence to create a Great Sphinx. Even greater intelligence is needed to create and sustain the natural wonders which surround us. It takes what we call Universal Intelligence. As humans, it's difficult for us to understand what it is, where it comes from or how it works. We know only that it must exist or nothing else would. There are some who equate Universal Intelligence to God. If that makes you comfortable, this theory works as well as any. One thing that is obvious, through both observation and logic, is that such an intelligence, by whatever name humans choose to call it, must exist.

For some, this idea is "unscientific." After all, one can't prove it or test it in a research laboratory. Yet, science is now expanding into areas such as quantum physics, and is welcoming fresh ideas. Scientists are even starting to accept the presence of a Universal Intelligence as a basic truth of the universe.

INNATE INTELLIGENCE

"Innate is an individualized portion of the ALL-WISE usually known as spirit."
— B.J. Palmer, D.C.

To chiropractors Innate Intelligence is not about how smart someone is—the level of a person's education or his or her ability to learn new material. A person with a Ph.D. in nuclear physics doesn't have any more Innate Intelligence than an aborigine who's never been out of the bush. Innate Intelligence guides us to adapt to our environment in order to survive. It allows nocturnal animals to have eyes that can see in the dark. It makes a leafy plant on a windowsill turn its leaves toward the light. Move the plant and it will turn its leaves again. You don't have to tell the plant what to do. The plant knows it has to have light to survive.

Obviously, the plant doesn't use logic to determine that it needs light. A plant doesn't think it all. Yet it knows how to use light, air and water and how to create a new plant. The plant knows what it has to do because it has Innate Intelligence.

Innate Intelligence makes a baby's heartbeat, digests food, eliminates waste, uses white blood cells to fight infections, and makes the baby cry when it wants attention. No one has to teach an infant any of these things.

THE TRIUNE OF LIFE

Of course, Innate Intelligence is the basis for proper function, but other factors are required for complete health.

If you were a master carpenter, you would be able to design a piece of furniture, draw out the pattern pieces, cut the wood, assemble the parts, and then stain and wax the finished piece. However, if you didn't have the pencil and paper to draw a pattern, or the tools to cut the wood and put it together, you could not make a cabinet. Or, if you had everything you needed, but lacked the strength to lift the hammer, you could not practice your craft.

Your Innate Intelligence is an expert in building a healthy body. But, if you don't have the proper energy, all the body parts or you are so weak physically and your body is in need of major repair, your body will not reflect health.

In chiropractic, strength is called Energy. The proper set of tools (all your body parts) is called Matter. These three elements, Innate Intelligence, Energy and Matter are known as the *Triune of Life*.

Living beings are like tiny universes. Each one is guided by a personal form of Universal Intelligence (Innate Intelligence) and also, each holds a mini-version of Universal Energy (Innate Energy).

"Chiropractors adjust subluxations, relieving pressure from the nerves so that they can perform their functions in a normal manner. The Innate can and will do the rest."
— B.J. Palmer, D.C.

VERTEBRAL SUBLUXATION, OR NERVE INTERFERENCE

If all three elements were always in perfect order, we would be in perfect health. Unfortunately, this is usually not the case.

In our world Innate Matter (our body) doesn't always function at peak performance. The brain sends messages to cells in the body, telling them what they need to do in specific parts of the body. Messages travel along a complex system of nerves. They can run into interference, some of the messengers may take detours, other slow down or lose their way.

Much of this interference occurs along the spine. This is the headquarters of the nervous system. All nerves from the brain travel down this road of interlocking bones, called *vertebrae*. They branch off and pass through openings along the spine to get to their destinations.

Occasionally, one or more of the vertebrae move out of alignment, we call this *nerve interference*, or a subluxation(s). Where misalignments occur, the spinal opening narrows, distorting the flow of Innate Energy throughout the body.

"The mysterious breakdowns of the body's intelligence… may be traceable to a single distortion—wrong detour…"
— Deepak Chopra, M.D.

If you have nerve interference, your body can't perform efficiently because it isn't getting the right messages from the brain.

Here's an example of what happens. When an unfriendly virus attacks, Innate Intelligence instructs the body to react and fight off the virus. This often means raising the body temperature so the fever can fight off the invader.

If the nerve flow is disturbed because of nerve interference, chemical imbalance occurs and the body will function less efficiently—its ability to fight off infection is diminished. If you experience one or more of the following symptoms: pain, dizziness, stiffness, weakness, profuse sweating, coughing, diarrhea, fever or stomach upset and vomiting, then it's time to receive an adjustment. Often these conditions are the result of one's body attempting to restore health. Correcting nerve interference will help your body return to normal function.

"To adjust the subluxation, then, is to advance mankind, step up his efficiency, increase his ability, make him more natural and more at peace with himself, for all things are possible to him who his body equals his Innate."
— B.J. Palmer, D.C.

Jonathan Falman's Experience

"My problem began quite unexpectedly. I bent down one day but couldn't stand straight again. At 57, I'm very active. I play a lot of tennis and my job as a mechanic at McDonald-Douglas requires me to bend and twist in some awkward positions, especially when I have to squeeze through the small openings in some of the jets I work on.

"Five days after the problem began; I was still suffering agonizing low back pain. I wasn't able to do anything.

"I took the recommendations of several friends and went to see a doctor of chiropractic who took x-rays. I was told that the problem was in my spine; and the doctors explained the spine's direct relation to my general health.

"When I came to the chiropractor, I couldn't even reach my knees with my hands. Now I can touch my toes without bending my knees, which I haven't been able to do for more years than I can remember. I can't thank my chiropractor enough."

We chiropractors work with the subtle substance of the soul. We release the prisoned impulses, a tiny rivulet of force, which emanates from the mind and flows over the nerves to the cells and stirs them to life. We deal with the magic power that transforms common food into living, loving, thinking clay; that robes the earth with beauty, and hues and scents the flowers with the glory of the air.

— B.J. Palmer

Chapter 3
Your Miraculous Body

The most amazing machine in the history of the natural world is the human body. If you were to purchase this machine it would cost millions of dollars. Once you brought it home you would treat it reverently. However special and valuable, we pay little attention to our body. In this chapter, I want to take you on a short tour of your body and remind you of its spectacular abilities. I want you to think about what would happen if there was interference to the nervous system that controls all body functions.

YOUR DNA—The Mastermind

The movie *Jurassic Park* has certainly illustrated how DNA contains the blueprint for life forms. The author of the novel (from which the movie was made), physician Michael Creighton, speculates that if it were possible to extract the DNA molecules of dinosaurs from amber containing fossilized remains, we could re-create these extinct creatures in today's world. Although it may be nothing more than a hypothetical theory, scientists have recognized the importance of DNA in identifying life forms.

Your body is made up of trillions of cells. Each cell contains DNA (deoxyribonucleic acid). A DNA molecule is so small that it requires an electron microscope to magnify it to be seen. It only takes one two-trillionth of an ounce of DNA to determine the kind of person you will be physically and mentally. In fact, the entire human race could be reproduced by an amount of DNA that would be equivalent to about the size of a dime.

When examined under a microscope, you can see that each DNA molecule contains atoms which are joined together to form a spiral. Unwound they would measure 5 feet in length! Since each of us begins with one cell, the DNA molecules in the single cell contain all the information needed to build your body. From how you look, to how your body works, all the designs are in your original DNA molecule. Every other cell in your body replicates the original molecule.

Even though there are about five billion people on the earth, each of us has different fingerprints and voice-prints. There are only eight basic fingerprint patterns but no two people have ever been found to have identical prints. Likewise, our voices are all unique. Each of us has a distinct energy wave pattern in our voice which can be charted by scientists. Interestingly enough, this pattern stays the same whether were shouting or whispering.

As you grow, your cells multiply by dividing over and

over again. These cells are so tiny that if you lined up four thousand of them, the line would only be one inch long. Cells come in many shapes and sizes depending upon their function.

They take in food and oxygen and eliminate waste. With the exception of brain cells, body cells are replaced by new cells upon completion of their life cycle. About every seven years the cells in the human body have completely been replaced. The reason you can remember things that happened long ago is that you keep your billions of brain cells all your life. They never die off, unless you destroy them.

YOUR BLOOD—The Stream of Life

Your blood is made up of billions of cells. It travels to your veins, arteries and capillaries on a stream of liquid called plasma. Innate Intelligence controls this flow of blood. The red cells carry oxygen from your lungs to your tissues.

They also take waste gas (carbon dioxide) out of the tissues and carry it back to your lungs where it can be exhaled. A red cell, which lives about four months, makes three thousand trips through your bloodstream. About ten million die off each minute, but with adequate nourishment new cells are quickly formed. Your body is constantly being bombarded by micro-organisms, which often get into the lymph fluid and are carried into the lymph nodes. Once they get there, your white cells(soldier cells), attack them. On any one day, there can be as many as thirty- to forty- billion soldier cells protecting you.

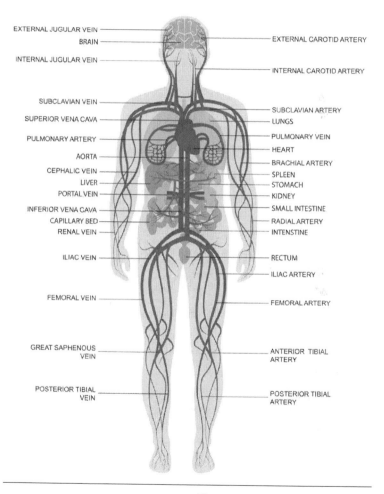

While these white cells are alive they fight off serious infections. Two-thirds of these cells are made in the marrow of your bones, as are all the red blood cells. They form a clot when you cut yourself, using fibrin to block off the opening and prevent the blood from flowing out of your body.

A drop of blood contains about five million red cells and seven thousand white cells, along with thousands of platelets (cells that are not red or white). Blood cells are very small—sixty thousand could be put on the head of a pin.

The average adult has four to six quarts of blood—about seven pounds or three-and-a-half quarts of blood for each one hundred pounds of body weight.

Blood is divided into four primary groups: Type O, which is the most common, Type A, Type B, and Type AB, which is the most rare.

YOUR HEART—The Pump

The heart is the strongest and toughest muscle in your body, weighing from nine to eleven ounces. The average heart beats about seventy-five times every minute. With each beat, it pumps blood into your lungs to pick up oxygen, and out of the lungs to supply the tissues in the body.   Both of these actions happen at the same time, even though you only feel one beat.

CIRCULATION OF BLOOD THROUGH THE HEART

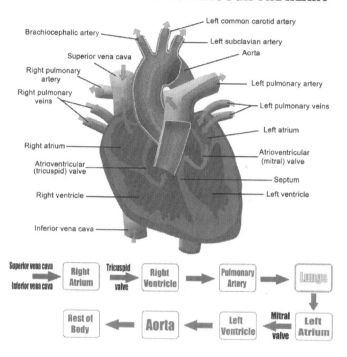

If you could track one blood cell, you would find it has been pumped throughout your entire circulatory system in sixty minutes. Stretched out end-to-end, your veins and arteries are about twelve thousand miles in length. It requires a strong muscle to pump blood through our bodies.

Normally, your heart pumps about two-and-a-half gallons of blood each minute. When you lie down, your heart slows down and you save about 824 beats each hour you rest. This gives your body more energy to fight disease.

YOUR LUNGS—The Bellows

If you've ever seen the way a bellow blows air to fan a fire, you have a pretty good idea of how the lungs work. *Alveoli* or air sacs surround the lungs which are made of a spongy tissue. Bronchial tubes penetrate the lungs, carrying the air you breathe to the single cell air sacs. Blood vessels wind around each sac. The molecules of oxygen leave the air in the sacs and pass into the blood. At the same time, carbon dioxide gas passes from the blood to the air sacs to be exhaled. The whole procedure of exchanging carbon dioxide for oxygen takes less than a second.

In the average twenty-four hour period, you will use about ninety gallons of pure oxygen or three thousand gallons of air. Your lungs are centered in your chest cavity, protected by your ribs, breastbone and diaphragm, which is a sheet of muscle at the base of your lungs.

It's the diaphragm that causes the lungs to expand and contract. As you breathe in, the diaphragm pulls down while your ribs and breastbone moves up.

Anatomy of Human Lungs

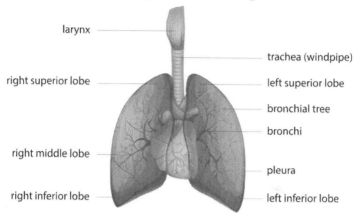

larynx

trachea (windpipe)

right superior lobe

left superior lobe

bronchial tree

bronchi

right middle lobe

pleura

right inferior lobe

left inferior lobe

This allows more room for the lungs to expand and fill with air. When you breathe out, the muscles relax and the air is expelled out of your lungs.

YOUR RESPIRATORY SYSTEM—The Filter

You wouldn't live very long if air went directly into the lungs without being filtered. Your lungs would fill up with dust, pollen, soot, spores, fibers and thousands of other particles floating in the air.

When you breathe, air enters your nose and passes through your windpipe into your lungs. The nasal passages are lined with a mucous membrane which is moist and covered with tiny hairs called cilia. The hairs and mucous trap dirt and germs, and keep them from entering your lungs. Your voice box, windpipe, and the thousands of small tubes in your lungs are covered with cilia. These continuously sweep away germs. Coughing and sneezing are innate safety devices to remove particles from your larynx and nasal passages.

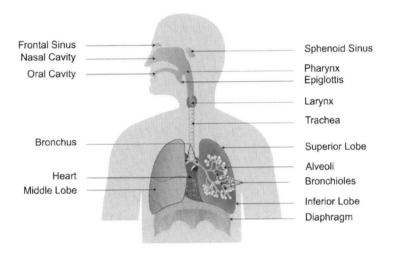

The mucus in your nose carries a germicide called lysozyme. This same germ-killing substance is found in your tears, and moves from your tear ducts into your nose to moisten and protect the nasal tissues.

> **"Innate knows more in one second than you can ever know."**
> — B.J. Palmer, D.C.

YOUR MUSCLES—Doing the Work

Each muscle consists of long, thin cells wrapped in bundles and held together by a tissue covering called the *fascia*. Some muscles are connected to tendons, which are strong white cords that anchor muscles to the bones. More than 600 muscles reside in your body, enabling you to perform even the simplest act.

There are three kinds of muscles. The *voluntary* muscles move when you cause them to. These are the muscles that you use to raise your arm or walk or turn your head. The *smooth* muscles operate without any conscious input from you. These include the muscles in the stomach, intestines and bladder. The heart is a muscle, too. It's made up of cells that look like tiny planks and it has more power than any other muscle in the body.

Muscles get their energy from oxygen, sugars and fat. They keep you warm by emitting heat. Muscles need activity. If you don't do something physical every day, your muscles can atrophy, and your general health will decline. See diagrams of the muscles on the next two pages.

Trapezius

Deltoid

Rhomboid

Teres Major

Triceps

Extensor Carpi Radialis

Extensor Carpi Ulnaris

Extensor digitorum

Extensor Digiti Minimi

Latissimus Dorsi

Thoraco-lumbar Fascia

Gluteus Maximus

Gracilis

Vastus Lateralis

Semimembranosus

Semitendinosis

Biceps Femoris

Gastrocnemius

Soleus

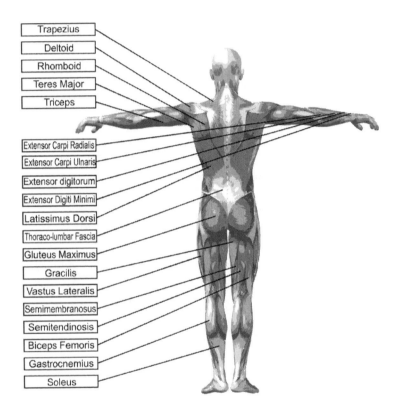

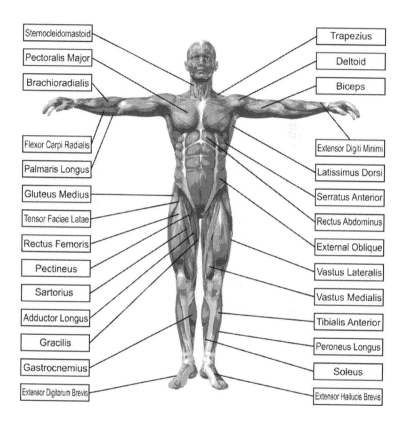

Sternocleidomastoid
Pectoralis Major
Brachioradialis
Flexor Carpi Radialis
Palmaris Longus
Gluteus Medius
Tensor Faciae Latae
Rectus Femoris
Pectineus
Sartorius
Adductor Longus
Gracilis
Gastrocnemius
Extensor Digitorum Brevis

Trapezius
Deltoid
Biceps
Extensor Digiti Minimi
Latissimus Dorsi
Serratus Anterior
Rectus Abdominus
External Oblique
Vastus Lateralis
Vastus Medialis
Tibialis Anterior
Peroneus Longus
Soleus
Extensor Hallucis Brevis

YOUR BRAIN – A Human Computer

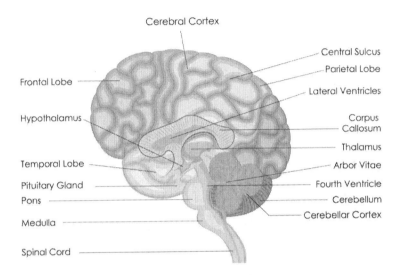

BRAIN

The human brain has the potential to be faster and store more information than any computer ever developed. Unfortunately, we have only learned to use a tiny percentage of our brain's capacity. Even so, your brain receives and interprets thousands of signals from every nerve in your body during every second of the day.

The largest part of the brain, the *cerebrum*, relays messages from the sensory organs, such as the nose, eyes, ears, tongue and skin, to the various parts of your body.

Certain areas of the cerebrum are responsible for specific functions, such as memory, reading comprehension, physical movement and so on. Another part of the brain, the *medulla oblongata*, controls automatic processes like breathing and keeping your heart beating. The *cerebellum*, is responsible for balance and motor coordination.

Your brain is connected to all parts of the body. The tail of the brain—the spinal cord emerges through an opening in the skull called the Foramen Magnum (a large hole.)

The spinal cord goes through the twenty-four bony rings or vertebrae, and the spinal nerves branch out from the various vertebrae to carry information to and from every part of the body. As stated before, when the nerves are impeded because the vertebrae are out of alignment, the result is a lack of normal function.

_____

YOUR STOMACH—The Food Processor

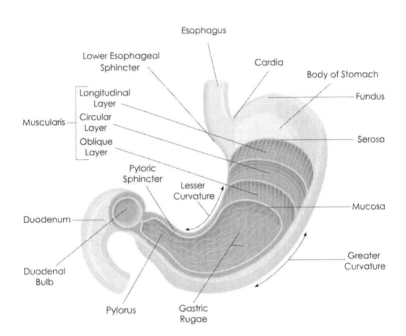

Stomach

Your stomach has amazing power. It can produce hydrochloric acid to break down the food you eat—an acid so strong that if put on your hand, blisters would appear.

Hydrochloric acid produces *pepsin* and *renin*, two other chemicals that prepare food to be digested by the intestines. The lining of the stomach is made of cells that produce tiny flakes of mucus. These line and protect the stomach, just like shingles protect the roof of a house.

Two-and-a-half quarts of gastric juices produced by your stomach each day allow you to digest a meal in one to seven hours, depending on what you have eaten. When the stomach is full, it contracts, helping to break down the food and push it towards the lower end of the stomach, the pylorus. From there, it goes into the intestines where all the nutrients are removed for use by the body and the waste is carried out of the body.

If you exercise immediately after you eat, or if you are very upset, you will slow down the digestive process and feel nauseated. Lack of food causes the stomach to contract in a rhythmic pattern, and we identify this as hunger pains.

YOUR SKIN—The Largest Organ of All

Although skin is only one-sixteenth to one-eighth inch thick, it has very important functions. The surface of the skin is called the *epidermis* and the layer below it is called the *dermis*. It is the epidermis that usually gets scraped when we skin a knee and unless we cut the dermis, we don't bleed. The lower layers of the epidermis contained a pigment called *melanin* which determines the skin color.

The more melanin you have, the darker your skin.

Your skin contains sweat and oil glands. Two million sweat glands allow you to excrete liquid waste material and stay cool through perspiration. The oil glands serve to waterproof your skin while keeping it from becoming too dry. The oil glands also keep your hair smooth and shiny.

Anatomy of Human Skin & Hair

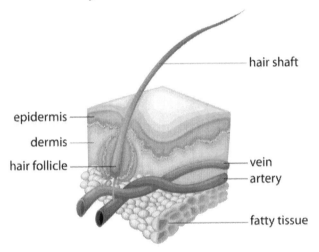

Blood circulates through your skin, helping to regulate body heat. If you get too hot, the blood vessels in your skin expand, coming closer to the surface of the skin where the outside air cools it. When you are cold, the blood vessels contract, so less blood is near the skins surface.

(NOTE: Exercise pushes blood near the surface of the skin. Fright moves it away.)

The *papillae* contain the nerves which connect the epidermis to the dermis and enable us to experience the sensation of touch.

Our skin doesn't wear away because new cells constantly renew the surface of the epidermis and the old cells die and flake away.

YOUR HANDS—The All-Purpose Tools

Have you ever taken the time to think about all the things you do with your hands? These really are remarkable tools that can distinguish size, shape, texture and temperature. They move, grasp or release objects, hold a pen to write, or play piano or stitch a fine seam.

The millions of tiny nerve endings send touch impulses to the brain which converts sensations into reactions and perceptions.

Just by touching a stove with your hand, your brain knows it is smooth and metallic, cool to the touch in some places and hot in others.

BONES OF THE RIGHT HAND

(OSSA MANUS)

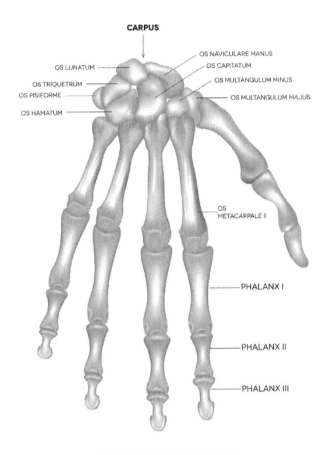

CARPUS

OS NAVICULARE MANUS

OS CAPITATUM

OS LUNATUM

OS MULTANGULUM MINUS

OS TRIQUETRUM

OS PISIFORME

OS MULTANGULUM MAJUS

OS HAMATUM

OS METACARPALE II

PHALANX I

PHALANX II

PHALANX III

FROM THE DORSAL SURFACE

lt

also knows that as your hand gets closer to the heat, you need to be careful you don't get burned.

The movements of your fingers are controlled by tendons—strong fibers that operate like a pulley cord to make the bones and muscles do what you want them to. The coordination between the tendons, muscles and bones is so perfect we are not even aware of it.

There are fifty-four bones in your hand; the thumb bone is the most versatile and the strongest. We tend to take our hands for granted, however, if deprived of the use of our hands, we would quickly realize how vital they are to everything we do.

YOUR FEET—Engineering Marvels

One-fourth of your body's bones are in your feet. Each foot contains twenty-six bones, linked together with thirty-three joints and attached by ligaments. The arch in your foot is an engineering marvel, built to withstand several hundred times its own weight and still keep the body balanced with mathematical precision. Five *metatarsal* bones are in each arch. They are attached to the *phalanges* or total bones at one end and the *tarsals* at the other. The tarsals connect the foot to the leg.

The arch distributes your weight evenly over your foot. If you weigh ninety-six pounds, the metatarsal bones attached to your big toes support eighty-eight pounds of your weight, and those attached to the smaller toes support your remaining eight pounds.

The average person walks about thirty thousand steps--twelve miles each day. At ninety-six pounds, you put 2,880,000 pounds of pressure on your feet in any twenty-four-hour period. And that's just walking! If you run, each step adds ten times your weight to your feet.

Bones of the Human Foot

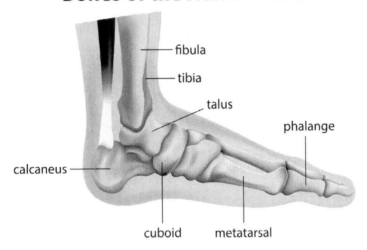

Because your feet are below your heart, the blood has to flow up from your feet against gravity. Inside your veins there are tiny gate valves which allow the blood to travel upward, preventing it from flowing back down and collecting in your feet.

(NOTE: When you experience an emotion like fear, the blood rushes to your brain and the temperature in your feet goes down. This is why we say someone "has cold feet" when they are afraid.)

The feet, like other parts of the body are truly amazing and wonderful mechanisms. It seems only Innate Intelligence could create such a remarkable living machine.

YOUR CHEMISTRY LAB—Your "24-Hour Drugstore"

"Medical men have searched the world for remedies, desiring an antidote. Chiropractors find the cause in the person ailing."
—B.J. Palmer, D.C.

Your magical chemistry lab supplies you with hundreds of chemicals to keep your body functioning properly. Chemicals keep your sinuses clear and your eyes working well; chemicals raise and lower your blood pressure and your body temperature; chemicals control your moods and help you digest your food and eliminate waste. There are also chemicals which guarantee your reproductive organs will work.

Your body also produces insulin and cortisone, and adrenalin and antibiotics, to fight infection—and this is only a fraction of the list. Science has much more to learn about the chemicals your body continually manufactures to keep you healthy.

Your magical chemistry lab includes specific instructions about how much of a chemical you need at any moment. It releases enough digestive juices to dissolve your stomach contents after a meal, and enough insulin to deal with the sugar you had in that piece of pie. If you're frightened, it will give you a shot of adrenaline to give you an extra boost of energy to take action. It releases clotting chemicals to the site of a wound and relaxants to allow you to get a good night's rest.

Your "laboratory" supplies everything to you at no cost. All it requires is that you give yourself the good care you deserve.

Your body is the most superb chemistry lab ever devised. It's as if you had the world's smartest health professional living inside you. Luckily our bodies work without any help from us. In fact, they work in spite of the mistreatment we often heap upon them.

Our Innate Intelligence controls every biological, chemical and physical action and reaction. When your Innate Intelligence is allowed to fully express itself, you have a better chance of reaching your maximum health potential. If you are functioning normally, every chemical you need will be delivered when it's needed, in the exact amount, twenty-four hours a day. It's a remarkably efficient system.

LACK OF PROPER CHEMICALS—Chaos

Timely delivery of chemicals to different areas of the body goes unnoticed but if delayed or canceled, the effect is often dramatic.

For instance, you can't hold a pen to write in less your brain produces a chemical called *dopamine,* which stimulates the basal ganglia and keep your extremities from shaking. A person with Parkinson syndrome is missing dopamine and can't thread a needle or hold a paper without shaking uncontrollably.

Chemicals ingested into the body often interfere with its natural action. For instance, you have a natural sleep cycle because your body produces the proper chemicals to allow you to sleep. However, if you drink a cup of coffee just before bedtime, the caffeine in the coffee may interfere with the chemical balance and sleep may elude you.

Sugar is a chemical that has adverse effects on the body—throwing it off balance. The famed pediatrician Lendon Smith, M. D., was asked to study a group of children who were considered hyperkinetic or hyperactive. He found they were routinely given the drug Ritalin to calm them down, but they turned into little zombies. However, after eating a heavily sugared meal they would again become very active.

Dr. Smith showed that the children's hyperkinetic behavior could be reversed by altering their diet and eliminating all the sugared breakfast cereals, lunchtime cake, mid-afternoon ice cream and before-bedtime candy.

Once children's sugar levels were brought under control, each child's pancreas didn't work overtime to produce enough insulin and the result for all that was a normal blood sugar level and modified behavior.

Your body doesn't want or need sugar. The body's chemistry lab isn't prepared to cope with it. And the result is all the unpleasant symptoms of high blood sugar hyperactivity or low blood sugar lethargy and depression.

Alcohol is another chemical that negatively affects our body. It creates, a chemical imbalance in the brain and alters peoples' behavior. Observe people who have had too many cocktails at a party. One person might be belligerent and hostile. Someone else might become loud and obnoxious, while another might become emotional and cry, or just fall into a stupor.

What we consider "normal" behavior is the result of *chemical balance*, which comes from well-functioning glands producing the chemicals at the command of the brain and spinal cord. The glands have a better chance of making the body function normally when there is no interference.

Nerve interference can bring all this "chemical laboratory" activity to a halt. Without any recognizable symptoms, your body's nerve supply may be interfered with causing your good health to change, depriving your body of the naturally produced chemicals to function properly, lowering your resistance and weakening your immune system.

Invest in your health; take time for regular check-ups. It's the best gift you can give yourself and your family.

The more you understand the way your body functions, the more you will be motivated to take care of yourself. Doctors of chiropractic are primarily interested in the proper function of body tissue and organs of the body—all controlled by the nervous system.

Chapter 4
Visiting a Chiropractor

Nerve interference has become a silent epidemic. Schedule a regular spinal check-up the way you schedule a routine dental check-up or a periodic eye exam. How long has it been since your spine was examined? For many people a scoliosis check in junior high was their last spinal examination.

When a chiropractor sees a new patient, it's common to find that muscles, ligaments, nerves, and internal organs are not in perfect order. The spine, too, often experiences some kind of degeneration.

THE PHYSICAL EXAMINATION

Your first visit will consist of a consultation and complete spinal examination. Most doctors will also provide some education if you're not familiar with chiropractic care.

"Chiropractors adjust the cause of dis-ease instead of treating the effects."
— B.J. Palmer, D.C.

The first thing you'll be asked to do when you visit a chiropractic office is fill out forms regarding personal information and health history. Then, the doctor will have a consultation with you and give you a chiropractic examination.

The most common examination is called palpation. The doctor carefully feels—or palpates—the entire spinal region to detect nerve interference. Other methods or instruments may be used to verify the findings. All of the examination techniques used by chiropractors are safe, painless and non-invasive.

Indications of nerve interference show up on an x-ray; soft tissue damage to nerves, muscles or discs—nerve impingement cannot be seen. For further diagnosis, some chiropractors utilize imaging tools such as MRIs, Thermography and Paraspinal EMGs and CT (CAT) scans. Your chiropractor will explain these methods in greater detail.

Use of x-rays should be a concern, but keep in mind that chiropractic does not use radiation as treatment or therapy, but only as a diagnostic tool. Chiropractic radiology generally exposes patients to a lot less radiation then similar orthopedic and medical examinations. Screens, shields, and high-speed x-ray film further reduce the danger of over exposure.

Chiropractors believe that the benefit must always justify the risks that are inherent; that's why we talk to our patients honestly, explain the risks, and answer questions in non-technical terms.

REPORT OF FINDINGS

After testing and diagnosis, you will receive a report of the doctor's findings. You'll be told if there is any nerve interference and how severe it is.

You and your doctor will discuss the health of your spine, and the doctor will outline a course of care needed to correct the nerve interference. This may include spinal adjustments, beneficial exercise and changes to your life-style.

Chiropractors don't treat symptoms. Our job is to locate the cause of dis-ease, the nerve interference, and correct it. Frequent adjustments may be required at the beginning of your treatment.

As your condition improves, the number of adjust-ments will decrease and you'll be placed on wellness care. Don't expect nerve interference to be corrected in a few visits. It will take continued adjusting to be certain the vertebrae have returned to their proper position, and to assure your muscles and ligaments can continue to hold them firmly in place.

Once you were properly "back together," your doctor will perform periodic spinal checks to make sure your spine remains free of nerve interference.

THREE LEVELS OF CHIROPRACTIC CARE:

There are three levels of chiropractic care.

First, is in Intensive Care Phase, Level I. During this time, the chiropractor's objective is to reduce stress damage to the spine and nervous system.

You might be in a situation where you have pain, or disease that has convinced you to seek help. Realize that the chiropractic adjustments are helping you immediately, but you have to understand healing takes time. Your condition didn't occur overnight. Be willing to change your personal habits and follow the doctor's advice to move the process forward.

During the Level I, you may be seeing your D.C. every day—or at least three times a week depending on the need.

Level II is the Reconstructive Phase. Now, the spine is nearly or completely aligned but it has to be monitored while it becomes stronger and holds the adjustment for longer periods of time. This stage is critical. Complete correction cannot take place if you don't have your spine checked regularly to be very sure there isn't a reoccurrence of nerve interference. During Level II, you may be seeing your chiropractor from one to two times a week.

Level III is the Wellness Phase. Now, your spine is holding its adjustment. This phase is similar to having your eyes checked or having your teeth cleaned. You want to visit your chiropractor on a regular basis. In this way, you can detect and correct nerve interference early, and enhance your body's Innate ability to express its maximum health potential.

PATIENT EDUCATION PROGRAMS

Unlike many other doctors, chiropractors don't work *on* our patients. We work *with* them. Health care and wellness care become a joint project for both the doctor and patient. To help educate the patients, most doctors offer some kind of information or educational program for new patients. This might consist of reading material, videotapes, a workshop, or orientation program.

If your D.C. offers a patient education program, take advantage of it. Read the material you receive. Watch the video tapes or listen to the audio tapes. Attend the presentations. Ask questions! The more you know and understand about chiropractic, the better able you'll be to help yourself.

Remember to visit your chiropractor even when you're under the care of a medical doctor. Medical doctors and other disciplines can't determine if you have nerve interference; they haven't been trained to recognize it. Your D.C. may help your body correct a condition naturally that an M.D. would treat with artificial chemicals or surgery.

"It is useless to administer a powder, potion, or pill to the stomach when the body needs an adjustment."
— B.J. Palmer, D.C.

PUT YOUR MIND AT REST

In 1994, the American Heart Association (AHA) gener-ated a great deal of publicity by announcing that re-searchers at the Stanford University School of Medicine had surveyed 486 California neurologists about the num-ber of patients they had treated in the preceding two years. Specifically, the researchers wanted to know about those patients who had suffered a stroke within twenty-four hours of cervical manipulation.

According to the AHA, the study showed that there was "small but significant risk" of a stroke occurring within twenty-four hours of cervical manipulation. The newspa-pers took the story and ran with it. Within days, headlines declared that *"Stroke Can Be Triggered by Twist of Neck, Study Claims."*

In every medium, the story was reported with sensa-tionalism. It was so slanted that chiropractors were put in the worst light imaginable—as if chiropractic and strokes were almost synonymous.

Have you ever read or heard about that article? Here's the truth:

- While 486 neurologists were questioned, (all of whom were in direct competition with chiroprac-tors) only 177 physicians responded and of those, only 37 claimed they had seen cases in which there might be a connection between cervical manipula-tion and the onset of a stroke.

- The study was a small one, never published, and not considered significant even by the researchers who set it up. Dr. Gregory W. Albers was one of the Stanford researchers. He said that the study "... was a small survey with a small sample size and it wasn't anything to make a big fuss over." He told me: "There's no question that probably most medical procedures carry a much greater risk—and there's no question what the leading causes of strokes are, and it's not chiropractic."

- Dr. Carlini said "... almost all interventions by allopathic physicians have a higher complication rate than chiropractic."

- As the benefits of chiropractic adjustments gain credibility, there are an increasing number of M.D.s, physical therapists (PT's), etc. who are attempting to train themselves in manipulation techniques at weekend seminars. This type of inadequate training presents a very real danger to the public's health, safety and welfare.

- Manipulation: "The forceful passive movement of a joint beyond its active limit of motion. It does not imply the use of precision, specificity, or the correction of nerve interference and, therefore, is not synonymous with the chiropractic adjustment."

- Adjustment: "The adjustment is the specific application of forces to facilitate the body's correction of nerve interference."

What we have is an all too common *leap of faith* by the media regarding an AHA article or study. Indeed, there has been the extremely rare occurrence of stroke following a cervical manipulation, but statistics show one stroke per several million. In any procedure, there is an element of risk because of the individual history of the patient, but statistically, your chance of dying from a bee sting or being killed by lightning is more likely.

Many of the stories I have heard have been hearsay and rumor, and have exploited the very rare occurrence of a stroke. You can be confident when you walk out of your chiropractor's office, after receiving an adjustment your overall health will be improved, not threatened.

Andrew Sanderson's Experience:

"About 30 years ago, I had a football injury. Over the next several years, I began to have pain in my left knee, a constant dull ache in the lower back on the right side and sinus trouble. I went to my medical doctors for help and they said I would have to live with this the rest of my life. The diagnosis was a permanently damaged nerve. The physicians suggested corrective surgery.

"I became very depressed. I couldn't sleep at night and I was very difficult to live with. I was going through hell and so was my family. It was then that I was convinced to try chiropractic. After my first few visits to my chiropractor, I felt a great deal of relief. Now I feel like a new person.

My back is greatly improved, without surgery, and it seems as if I never even had knee problems or sinus trouble. It changed my life. When you feel good, you look good, and you develop a healthy attitude. It wasn't very long before everyone noticed the great improvement in me. My only regret is that I waited so long!"

Doctors of Chiropractic are committed to patient education. Patients appreciate knowing, in advance, the value and purpose of every procedure before it is rendered. Ask questions and get involved!

Chapter 5
Here's to Your Health

I've discussed the body's ability to heal itself—the army of white blood cells, anti-bodies, leukocytes, mast cells, neutrophils and eosinophils. They are internal antibiotic soldiers which patrol and protect every inch of the body from injury and infection.

Even when the body organism is hosting a serious condition, we still have the capacity to heal a cut or overcome an infection.

Medical journals constantly print stories of patients who have recovered spontaneously from incurable illness. Patients who have been given six months to live, are still telling the story thirty years later. There's no definite answer to why this happens.

No one understands spontaneous remission, but all healthcare professionals acknowledge that we carry within us a miraculous ability to heal ourselves.

Given our body's ability to heal itself, why do we get sick? Why don't we heal ourselves every time? There are genetic factors we don't understand that strongly affect how are Innate Wisdom works to heal us. It's the mission of every chiropractor to help patients raise their natural and Innate healing ability to its highest potential.

Chiropractic's main concern is not with the trauma that follows accidents, most of which is emergency first aid—setting bones, stitching wounds closed, and removing foreign objects. That is your medical doctor's job. This is an example of how two divergent healthcare philosophies can complement each other and forge a cooperative effort.

Unfortunately, other problems are often handled with drugs. These dangerous, artificial chemicals are dispensed to control the symptoms—lower the fever, kill germs and deaden pain. Instead of correcting the underlying cause, these warning signals are ignored, and healing is actually delayed.

Our society is full of people who are little more than walking medicine cabinets. They take handfuls of pills throughout the day. Instead of finding out and correcting what is causing the high blood pressure, they take medicine to lower it. Instead of determining the underlying metabolic reason for their condition, they rely on artificial chemicals for a temporary cover-up. If they stop taking the medicine, the condition returns. This isn't health and healing. This is containment and control.

As a chiropractor, I believe that at the root of many of these conditions is nerve interference. This isn't to say that if your spine is healthy, you'll never have a sick day and you'll live forever. No one can promise you that. We come into the world marked "terminal," because as human beings we all die. However, without nerve interference, you can be confident you have a better chance for a longer healthier existence.

THE NEUROLOGICAL BASIS OF DISEASE

If you are still unclear about the connection between the spine and overall health, you need to know the story of Masha and Dasha Krivoshlyapova, one of the most unusual sets of co-joined twins ever born. When they were born, on January 4, 1950, their mother was told they had died shortly after birth. In fact, they had been taken to a Soviet institution near Moscow for study, observation and experimentation. For nearly forty years, they were isolated from their family and the world.

Co-joined (Siamese) twins result when a single fertilized egg doesn't split completely, as it does in the case of identical twins. Instead the egg remains joined at some point and the children are born partially attached. Usually, these children are spontaneously aborted as embryos, but on rare occasions, they are born alive. If the connection isn't extensive, they can sometimes be separated successfully. In a 1993 case, one twin was sacrificed so her sister, the stronger of the two, could have a chance to live.

In the case of Masha and Dasha, the co-joining was so extensive that an operation to separate them would've killed them both. It was the unique way in which they were joined that caused the Soviet scientists to be so interested in them.

The girls were born with four arms and three legs. They stood on two legs, one controlled by each twin, and a vestigial third leg remained in the air behind them. It's not surprising that it took them until they were five years old before they developed the coordination to be able to walk.

Their upper intestines were separate, but they shared a lower intestine and rectum. They had four kidneys and one bladder and one reproductive system. From the waist up, they were two distinct persons with interconnected circulatory systems, so they shared each other's blood. When a virus entered one sister's bloodstream, it soon appeared in the other sister's blood as well. However, illness affected them quite differently. In fact, in an interview in 1989, Masha complained they had always been treated as one person when their medical files were quite diverse.

For instance, Dasha was near-sighted, caught cold easily and was right-handed. Masha, who was left-handed, smoked occasionally but still had a stronger constitution than her sister, even though she had slightly higher blood pressure.

The question that puzzled scientists was why one sister would get measles and the other wouldn't, even though the germ was in both of their bodies. Russian pathologist, A.D. Speranski, realized that the nervous system had a definite role in the development of disease. The healthier the nervous system, the more the body could fight off illness. In the case of Masha and Dasha, what was it that caused one to be sick and the other to stay well?

The answer became apparent. While they shared their circulatory, digestive, excretory, lymphatic, and endocrine
system and had a common skeletal system from where they were joined at the hips, they had separate spinal columns and skulls. They had separate spinal cords and separate brains. This was the only significant difference between them!

These remarkable twins lived their lives as a walking laboratory in which scientists verified that disease and sickness do indeed have a neurological basis. Because of them, researchers have proved one can't get sick simply from being exposed to germs. One's body has to supply those germs with a fertile breeding ground where they can multiply and grow. That's why one twin could be ill when the other wasn't.

Each of us breathes in millions of germs every time we inhale, and we breathe out even more germs when we exhale. If the cause of illness were as simple as being exposed to bacteria, we would all be sick all the time.

One last note about Masha and Dasha. In 1989, they were released from the institution, rejoined their mother and were looking forward to a happier future. However, as distressing as the first forty years of their lives were, they could take some comfort in the knowledge that they have significantly advanced our understanding of how the brain and spine affect our general health.

THE ADJUSTMENT

At the heart of chiropractic care is the adjustment. A spinal adjustment is a specific application of forces used to facilitate the body's correction of nerve interference. The force must be given with the right amount of pressure in the proper direction at the right time. While it is usually done with the doctor's hands, adjusting instruments are used too.

We often hear that patients believe there are different adjustments for different conditions. They think there is a specific adjustment for high blood pressure that is different from the adjustment for a headache. The adjustment has one purpose and one purpose only—to correct or reduce nerve interference. The potential healing of a symptomatic condition or disease often results from the correct nerve flow to the affected area and improvement of your overall body chemistry. Remember, the symptom is usually the warning signal to alert you that something is wrong.

If you don't have any symptoms and visit your chiropractor as part of a wellness program, you won't receive an adjustment unless you have nerve interference. Having a disease, or other health condition, won't warrant an adjustment unless you have nerve interference.

"In the future, chiropractic will be valued for its preventative qualities as much as for relieving and adjusting the cause of ailments."
— B.J. Palmer, D.C.

What you can expect from your adjustment is a feeling of peace and relaxation that can last from a day to a week. Patients often comment that they experience a better night's sleep and increased energy. It's common to hear that they went home and tackled that project they've been putting off for months.

Some patients report that their symptoms start to go away after the first adjustment, while others don't feel any immediate difference. If you don't feel a change, don't be discouraged. Often you are not aware of internal improvements.

Some patients may feel discomfort after their first adjustment, ranging from a headache to just general fatigue. In almost every case, this feeling goes away within the next couple adjustments.

This discomfort is often due to a detoxification of the body after adjustments. As poisons leave the system, they could create a headache or slight head cold, even a slight fever and a feeling of lethargy.

Muscles may become sore after being adjusted. You may feel soreness like you had a workout at the gym. This condition is always temporary and disappears as your muscles gain strength and flexibility.

Spinal nerves that have been impinged and stressed for many years are suddenly coming back to life. These changes are exciting! As they heal, they become sensitive, and the old injury pains may return during a necessary and beneficial body phenomenon called "retracing." During "retracing," the healing process is repeated as if the injury had happened yesterday, instead of possibly years before.

If your response to an adjustment is euphoria, it's most likely because the newly freed nerves are sending Innate Energy through the opened passages and releasing the physical stress you've become accustomed to feeling. Life is being turned on.

If you feel little change, it may be that your general health is very good—the nerve interference was caught at an early stage before much damage occurred. Each of us is different, and no two of us react the same. But everyone will benefit from the correction of nerve interference.

RETRACING

Chiropractors have found that body tissues have a memory which records and holds onto the traumas, injuries and accidents it has experienced. Along with the memory of physical pain, the body also recalls the feelings of fright, shock, or anger and hysteria that accompanied the trauma. When the patient begins healing after an adjustment, it is possible to re-experience some discomfort from an old injury. If this happens, patience is needed to work it through.

Although, retracing is often low-key and almost unnoticeable, it can be dramatic for a short time. When it is intense, the patients may feel worse instead of better. Unfortunately, if the patient isn't prepared for this reaction, he or she may terminate the care and cheat themselves out of recovery.

The idea of retracing is used in several branches of healing. John Upledger, Doctor of Osteopathy, calls retracing *unwinding*. Homeopathy refers to it as *flashbacks,* and states that according to the three-part healing process called Hering's Law, cures occur first, from the inside to the exterior; second, from the most vital to the least vital; and third, in reverse order from how the symptoms appeared.

Psychologists recommend *re-scripting* in order to come to terms with unpleasant past experiences. Re-scripting involves working through past history and rewriting it to have the outcome you wanted.

Typical examples of retracing which occur on the path of healing might be the return of original symptomatic pain after several adjustments. While the pain can be severe, it usually clears up quickly.

These are further examples of how our body strives to heal itself in ways we don't fully understand.

TIME TO HEAL

One of the first questions many chiropractic patients ask is, "How long is this going to take?" This is a question they may not think to ask a medical doctor. Some drug treatments are prescribed for a lifetime. The chiropractor cannot be expected to undo years of dis-ease in a single visit. It just doesn't work that way.

Your doctor will try to tell you how long it might take before you achieve maximum correction. Whatever the answer, it will be based on three considerations.

First, the doctor will look at the objective results of any diagnostic instrumentation, or tests, and your physical examination. **Second,** the doctor will assess the experience with other patients who had similar nerve interference patterns. **Third,** he or she will consider those characteristics that are unique to you, including your age, how long you've had your nerve interference, your general health history, genetic factors, emotional stress and diet.

The secret is to be patient. Work with your doctor, and be very honest about how feel about your care. The better your relationship with your chiropractor—the better your total healing experience.

"Why search the world over for an exterminator or an antidote for dis-ease? Why not look for the cause of the ailments in the person affected and then correct it?"
— B.J. Palmer, D.C.

"I'D RATHER DO IT MYSELF!"

Have you ever bent over and heard your spine snap, crackle and pop like a bowl of breakfast cereal? Have you ever gotten out of bed in the morning and moved in exaggerated gestures to make your body create popping sounds, after which you felt immeasurably better for awhile? Have you ever thought you didn't need to see a chiropractor because you could do an adjustment on yourself?

Every doctor has, at one time or another, been at a social function where someone wants to demonstrate how easy it is to "crack" themselves. They proceed to assume a variety of positions that cause large popping sounds to emanate from their spine. "See," they say triumphantly, "how hard is it to do that?"

The truth is, the more you can stretch your spine, the healthier your spine will be. Spinal exercises or stretches, like yoga, are good for you and will probably make you feel better. However, if the vertebrae aren't moving when your spine is "popping" from the stretches, they will continue to make cracking sounds until your doctor has been able to adjust the cause of your nerve interference and correct it. Only your chiropractor knows the exact technique and force necessary to correct your nerve interference.

It's also possible that you have a misalignment which is beneficial. Sometimes, the body has to misaligned the vertebrae in order to prop up a weakened area of the spine. These are called compensatory or defensive mis-alignments. The doctor of chiropractic will recognize that and not attempt to change it. It takes expertise to determine the difference between compensatory misalignment and nerve interference. If you or a well-meaning friend play around with spinal manipulation, you can cause real harm if you further weaken an area that's already in trouble.

One other word of caution: occasionally we hear of someone who was paralyzed, and after falling out of a wheelchair, suddenly could walk. It's true, that in rare instances there is an accidental adjustment that restores mobility to people who have been afflicted with limited mobility for months or years. However, these instances are so rare that they are usually well-publicized when they occur. When it happens, it's magical. But don't assume it's going to happen to you. Statistically, you'd have a better chance of winning the lottery. Instead, call the chiropractor and have your spine checked out so you can be your best every day.

"While other professions are concerned with changing the environment to suit the weakened body, chiropractic is concerned with strengthening the body to suit the environment."
— B.J. Palmer, D.C.

Everyday scientists and researchers are proving what doctors of chiropractic have known since 1895.

Chapter 6
A Chiropractor's Education

Two years after discovering the benefit of chiropractic care, D.D. Palmer opened the first chiropractic college. It was 1897 in Davenport, Iowa, when the Palmer Infirmary and Chiropractic Institute opened its doors. Less than a century later, there are eighteen chiropractic colleges in the United States and eight in six foreign countries.

Chiropractic education is every bit as comprehensive as is medical education. Before being accepted by a chiropractic college, students must have completed a minimum of two years of undergraduate work with a heavy emphasis on basic sciences.

Once in Chiropractic College, the four-year course of study is longer than that required of most medical students. In addition to classroom and lab work, each student chiropractor must complete a period of internship during which students care for patients under the close supervision of instructors. This is often followed by an *ex*-ternship program during which students assist field chiropractors in their offices. Since these students don't yet have degrees and licenses, they don't adjust spines. As students, they are there to assist, observe and learn.

CHIROPRACTIC COMPARED TO MEDICAL EDUCATION		
	CHIROPRACTIC Classroom Hours	**MEDICAL** Classroom Hours
Anatomy	540	508
Physiology	240	326
Pathology	360	401
Chemistry	165	325
Microbiology	120	114
Diagnosis	630	324
Neurology	320	112
X-Ray	360	148
Psychiatry	60	144
Obstetrics	60	148
Orthopedics	210	156
Total Hours	**3,065**	**2,706**

This comparison chart is based on the review of curriculum catalogs from eleven chiropractic colleges and twenty-two medical schools in the United States. It clearly shows that chiropractors are among the best-trained health practitioners you can find.

Please note that chiropractic schools study both geriatrics and pediatrics, while eye, ear, nose, throat and dermatology are combined with diagnosis.

After students have acquired the necessary foundation of knowledge during the early part of their schooling, they later focus on specialized subjects, including chiropractic philosophy and practice, along with chiropractic diagnosis and adjusting techniques that aren't taught in any other healthcare field.

Before obtaining their degrees, all students must complete approximately nine hundred hours of work in the clinic setting. Because chiropractic students don't have to spend time studying pharmacology or surgery, as their medical counterparts do, they are given additional training in anatomy, nutrition, diagnosis, palpation, x-ray, and a variety of adjusting techniques. In fact, chiropractic students log more educational hours in these subjects then their medical counterparts.

After new chiropractors have graduated, they must then pass a state license exam in any state where they wish to practice. Most graduates take the National Board of Chiropractic Examination which tests the doctors' knowledge in many areas. These particular tests are so comprehensive that most states now accept them as the state license exam. In addition, a Doctor of chiropractic must also pass a practical exam and interview conducted by the State Board of Chiropractic Examiners in the state where they are seeking a license.

Cause and Cure

"A cause must be adjusted, corrected, fixed. To cure, you must treat effects, apply something to the results. Therein lies the greatest transforming value of chiropractic; it adjusts causes, but does not treat effects."

— B.J. Palmer, D.C.

Eleanor Drusart's Experience

"I first injured my back twenty years ago, and I've been having back trouble off and on ever since. The last four years, I've been having muscle spasms in my back which became more frequent and progressively worse. I had constant headaches, and was irritable, nervous, tired and depressed, and I had not had my period for the last four years. An orthopedic doctor I had been seeing recommended surgery but couldn't guarantee it would help.

"Because I'm a nurse, I rejected the idea of going to a chiropractor. Instead, I just suffered, spending several days in bed with painkillers, a taped-up back and a heating pad. Finally, I was in constant pain and couldn't take it anymore. One day, several friends told me of the help they received from their chiropractor, so I made an appointment to see him that very day. That's when I had my miracle.

"After my first adjustment, I left the office and got in my car to leave. Without any warning I started my menstrual cycle. This may sound incredible but that's what happened. I no longer have any muscle spasms or back pain. I'm doing things I haven't done in years. I don't take pain-killers or tranquilizers since I started my adjustments. I really enjoy living again! I hope someday chiropractors work as an integral part of the medical profession."

Chapter 7
Your Child and Chiropractic

Every baby needs to have a healthy spinal column. It's the framework that will support your child throughout his or her growing years and adulthood. Studies have shown that newborn infants often enter the world with spinal trauma due to the birth process. Even under the best conditions, birthing can be difficult for the infant who has spent nine months cradled in the dark, warm "waterbed" of the womb. It's very important to have your infant checked by a chiropractor shortly after his or her birth to be certain that there isn't any nerve interference. Periodic checks should continue throughout your child's lifetime.

Robert S. Mendelsohn, M.D., was one of America's leading pediatricians and a vocal proponent of home delivery. In his consciousness-raising book, *Confessions of a Medical Heretic,* he discussed how babies born in the hospital are six times more likely to suffer distress during labor and delivery, eight times more likely to get caught in the birth canal, four times more likely to need resuscitation, four times more likely to become infected, and thirty times more likely to be permanently injured.

A study conducted by Luis E. Mehl, M.D., of the University of Wisconsin Infant Development Center reviewed two thousand births. Nearly half of these had been home deliveries. Fourteen of the home-born babies had to be resuscitated, as compared to fifty-two of those born in the hospital. And only one home-delivered baby suffered neurological damage compared to six of the hospital born babies.

The figures reveal the benefits of home delivery. This is why many chiropractors and their families select natural childbirth at home.

In 1987, the German medical journal, *Manuelle Medizin,* published a report of a study which examined 1250 babies five days after birth. Of this group, 211 suffered from vomiting, hyperactivity and sleeplessness. Upon examination 95 percent of these children had spinal abnormalities. After being adjusted, all the infants became quiet, the crying stopped, their muscles relaxed and they went to sleep.

The same report said that they found over one thousand infants with nerve interference in the upper neck area, which caused a variety of clinical conditions, ranging from central motor impairment to lowered resistance to infections—especially those of the ears, nose and throat.

In one case history, an eighteen-month-old boy suffered from tonsillitis, frequent enteritis, conjunctivitis, colds and earaches. Because of all these ailments he had trouble sleeping. After his first spinal adjustment, the little boy began to sleep through the night, and it wasn't long before he was in good health.

Scientists are still learning how to accurately assess the damage to infants. They do know that a slight pull on the neck during delivery can cause a subluxation that might cause damage too slight to be noticeable immediately. But eventually it might cause some learning disability.

One of the greatest gifts you can give your newborn is a complete spinal examination by a doctor of chiropractic.

CHIROPRACTIC FOR CHILDREN

Chiropractors feel strongly that the entire family can benefit by having spinal checkups.

The children who have been under regular chiropractic care get sick less often and less severely. They rarely miss days from school. Recent studies have also shown that they have fewer emotional and learning disabilities and other neurological problems connected with childhood.

In 1989, a study compared the patients of two hundred pediatricians with two hundred children who had been under the care of chiropractors. Not only was the overall health of the chiropractic children superior to those who had known only medical treatment, but they also had fewer ear infections, fewer allergies, lower incidence of tonsillitis and less need to be given antibiotic therapy.

EAR INFECTIONS

Every parent has been awakened at sometime during the night by the sound of a child crying from the agony of an ear infection. Usually, the culprit is a very painful condition called *acute otitis media*. The fever soars to 103 degrees or higher and fluid oozes out of the ear.

Most pediatricians will treat and ear infection with an antibiotic such as ampicillin or penicillin or an oral decongestant. Putting tubes in the ears and surgery on the eardrum (myringotomy) are used in severe cases. The problem is that every one of these treatments has negative side effects.

In the book, *How to Raise a Healthy Child . . . In Spite Of Your Doctor*, Dr. Robert S. Mendelsohn cites a double-blind study in which 171 children with acute otitis media were divided into four groups. The severity of the condition ranged from one ear to both ears being infected.

The first group received myringotomy surgery. The second group was given antibiotics. The third group was given a combination of surgery and antibiotics, and the fourth group received no chemical or surgical treatment at all. The authors of the study found that there was no significant difference between the four groups in terms of pain, temperature, discharge, otoscopic appearances or hearing loss. Furthermore, no one group suffered recurrences more than any other. In short, recovery was about the same for everyone, whether or not anything had been done.

Another study revealed that when antibiotics are given for ear infections, especially on the first day of the onset of infection, the disease isn't shortened by any measurable clinical standard. Antibiotics not only fail to cure the problem, but they fail to prevent recurrence as well. In fact, recurrence rates were higher in children treated with antibiotic therapy.

And other common treatment for ear infections, mentioned previously, is a tympanotomy which is a surgical procedure that inserts a two in the ear of a child. This operation is so common it is performed over 1.2 million times each year.

A British study examined patients who had received the tube in one ear but not in the other. Researchers showed that the eardrum with the tube tended to develop scar tissue that have the potential of leading to future hearing loss while the untreated ear healed normally without any problem. Although chiropractic doesn't treat ear infections, when a chiropractor corrects nerve interference, it often corrects a chemical imbalance, inviting the body to respond with its own powerful immune system. An eighteen-year study of 4600 cases of upper respiratory infections in a core group of one hundred families found that when spinal motion was restricted in the upper neck area, ear infection occurred. When spinal motion was maintained or re-established, complication usually didn't develop.

If your children have ear infections, chances are they have nerve interference, and you need to get them to a chiropractor for adjustments. When you do this, there is a good chance you will promote better health and also be able to avoid adverse drug reactions, side effects and allergic responses from medical treatments.

TONSILS AND ADENOIDS

The tonsils are a very important part of the human immune system. They are too small lymph glands that sit at the back of the throat to protect us from infection and disease. When the body fights infection, the tonsils can become enlarged and inflamed and covered with a white material. This condition, tonsillitis, is very painful. If tonsillitis is part of an upper respiratory infection, it's accompanied by a mild fever, cough, congestion and a runny nose. If it's the result of strep bacteria, there is a higher fever, the lymph glands in the neck become swollen and tender, and the breath may have a foul odor.

The adenoids are also lymph glands in the throat which fight disease. Unlike the tonsils, they are out of sight but they also serve to protect us from disease.

For several decades, tonsillectomies were one of the most common operations of childhood with one-and-a-half to two million being performed each year. In fact, there was a time when they were removed as just one of the "rights of passage." Unfortunately, the vast majority of the tonsillectomies were unnecessary. The only reason to ever remove adenoids or tonsils is because of a malignancy or airway obstruction caused by the tonsils swelling to the point where they have closed the throat and the child can't breathe. Any other reason for surgery is dangerous to your child's health.

Children's tonsils were most often removed to reduce the incidence of sore throat. However, sore throats involve a virus, not bad tonsils. Removing the tonsils may pose more danger to the child's health. When the tonsils are gone, so is the child's first line of defense against infection. Now, the burden of fighting disease is transferred to the lymph nodes in the neck, which can lead to more dangerous complications.

Chiropractors know that it's perfectly normal for the body to host a certain amount of bacteria in the throat area without becoming ill. When your children are free from nerve interference, they will be better able to maintain a high level of natural immunity. A 1976 study showed that seventy of seventy-six children suffered from restricted movement in the upper neck area. Adjustments which resulted in correction of nerve interference allowed the children to fight off infection naturally and return to good health without complication.

SCOLIOSIS

At some time during the early school years, almost every parent is asked to give permission for his or her child to have a scoliosis exam. Normally, everyone's spine curves slightly to the right or left and may even have vertebrae that manifest a little twisting or rotation. *Scoliosis is an excessive curve or twist of the spine.*

In most cases, the cause of scoliosis is unknown. Only ten-to-fifteen-percent of scoliosis cases can be traced to a tumor, infection, cerebral palsy, muscular dystrophy, disc problems or birth deformity.

Scoliosis isn't a terminal condition, and most people can lead a perfectly normal life without ever knowing they have it. In rare cases, where the scoliosis is more than 30 degrees, there may be impaired respiratory or heart function that's thought to be neurological in origin rather than mechanical.

The orthodox medical approach to scoliosis has undergone some changes. Before 1945, the body was encased in a plaster cast. Then doctors surgically used rods and metal restraints to straighten the spine. Other brace devices followed and then, electrical stimulation therapy became popular. Surgeons were quoted as saying that none of these methods did any good whatsoever. The newest research claims that 95 percent of all scoliosis patients can be identified by neurological tests, indicating the problem originates in the nervous system. Since chiropractors correct nerve interference, the best answer to the problem of scoliosis is to allow a chiropractor to adjust the vertebrae to correct the nerve interference which has caused or aggravated the condition.

LEARNING DISORDERS

Current statistics indicate that eight million school children in the United States have a learning impairment, which can be traced back to some sort of malfunction in the nerve system.

When children have trouble learning, their frustration adversely affects their relationship with everyone around them—parents, siblings, teachers and school mates. Often, when a child develops a self-esteem problem, he or she is prone to emotional problems and psychological impairments that may carry into adulthood.

When children are hyperactive, due to emotional problems, medical treatment often includes medication, such as the drug, Ritalin, which has severe side effects. Ritalin doesn't always work and it often does more harm than good.

Recently, the director of Psychoeducational and Guidance Services of College Station, Texas, noted that out of 10,000 hyperactive children referred to him in the preceding decade, those who showed the most improvement had received chiropractic care. This caused the organization to refer some students to chiropractors for adjustments so they could monitor the effect of the care. Out of twenty-four students who had learning impairments, twelve received chiropractic care and the remaining students either received medication or no treatment at all.

The study concluded that chiropractic was 20 percent

to 40 percent more effective than the better-known medications. Because students who are seriously afflicted seem to benefit so well from chiropractic, it seems inescapably logical that a "normal" child would benefit as well. It follows that chiropractic care can help an average student become above average. Perhaps a child's I.Q. can be raised—reading skills improved, as well as being given an edge in alertness, coordination and speech.

"Chiropractors correct abnormalities of the intellect as well as those of the body."
— D.D. Palmer

CAN IT HELP MY CHILD?

"He knows when it flows above down, from inside out, naturally from the brain to the body, we are healthy and well."
— B.J. Palmer, D.C.

We recommend all children be checked regularly for nerve interference, even without symptoms present.

However, if you know a child who is not under chiropractic care, and suffers from any of the following problems, please urge the child's parents to consider chiropractic.

- Fever
- Colic
- Croup
- Allergies
- Wheezing
- Poor posture
- Stomach ache
- Hearing loss
- Neck/back pain
- Leg/hip/foot pain
- Numbness

- Headaches
- Cough/colds
- Asthma
- Bedwetting
- Bronchitis
- Constipation
- Weakness/fatigue
- Ear infections
- Skin problems
- One leg shorter
- Irritability

- Neck aches
- Nervousness
- Learning disorders
- Sinus problems
- Eye problems
- Scoliosis
- Arthritis
- Fatigue
- Pain in joints
- Shoulder/arm pain
- Poor concentration

Parents who are aware of the importance
of a properly functioning nerve system
automatically want their children
checked by a doctor of chiropractic.

Chapter 8
Chiropractic and the Elderly

Americans are living longer than ever before. In addition to living into our 80s and 90s, we are more active than we used to be.

The study of geriatrics shows that it's possible to live a long, full life, and perhaps slow down the aging process.

Seniors can improve their strength, too. Dr. Maria Fiatarone affiliated with Tufts University and Harvard Medical School conducted a study in which nine seniors, ranging in age from eighty-six to ninety-six, worked out with a weight machine three times a week. They increased the strength of their quadriceps by an average of 174 percent. As one 92-year-old woman said: "They made a new person out of me."

Not only is physical health maintainable, but so is mental health. In his best-selling book, *Quantum Healing*, Deepak Chopra states that:

"Careful study of healthy elderly people... has revealed that 80 percent of healthy Americans, barring psychological distress (such as loneliness, depression or lack of outside stimulation), suffer no significant memory loss as they

age.
The ability to retain new information can decline... but the ability to remember past events, called long-term memory, actually improves. As long as a person stays mentally active, he/she will remain as intelligent as in youth and middle age."

WHAT EXTENDS LIFE?

Gerontologists, scientists who study aging, now feel that life should continue to 100 or even 120 years, but they are surprised that so few make it. In 1995, the oldest woman in the world celebrated her 120th birthday and it was considered an unusual event around the world. While some centenarians are found to be drinkers and smokers, others shun tobacco and alcohol. Some are meat eaters and others are vegetarians. They can be religious or atheists. Many have led relatively easy lives, and there are some who have encountered tremendous difficulties. No one is quite certain what the magic ingredient is.

Studies have shown that the chances for longevity increase when people follow a low-fat, low cholesterol, vegetarian diet and keep physically and mentally active. Furthermore, the subjects of these studies only visit a medical doctor on rare occasions.

THE MEDICAL APPROACH

Statistics show that there are 42.3 million people aged sixty and over living in the United States. Of these older adults, 9.6 million experience adverse reactions to prescribed and over-the-counter drugs every year. These reactions include drug-induced car accidents and falls, memory loss, Parkinsonism, ulcers and death, from overdoses of heart medicines and anesthetics. In 1991, people in this age group filled 650 million prescriptions—an average of slightly more than fifteen prescriptions per person.

In their book, *Worst Pills, Best Pills II*, Sydney M.Wolfe, M.D. and Rose-Ellen Hope, R.Ph., of the Public Citizen Health Research Group, expose the severe overmedication of our older citizens. Forty to fifty percent of the medications were overused and mis-prescribed, especially tranquilizers (including sleeping pills and mindaltering drugs), cardiovascular drugs and gastrointestinal drugs. The medications that are used to treat heart disease, high blood pressure and vascular disease were found to be the most abused.

Older adults make up one-sixth (16.7%) of the population. This 16.7% of the population uses:

- 33.3% of all tranquilizers
- 50% of all sleeping pills
- 33.3% of all antidepressants
- 65% of all high blood pressure drugs
- 84% of all blood vessel dilating drugs
- 43% of all gastro-intestinal drugs

- 20% of all cold, cough, allergy, and asthma drugs
- 33% of all arthritis drugs

Many older adults are happy to take medication to relieve their aches and pains. The medical community and the drug industry, has also led them to believe these drugs will extend their lives.

Doctors often share the belief that an office visit should end by writing a prescription for an elderly patient. They may not know a great deal about geriatric medicine and they may fail to realize the danger drugs may have on these adults. Too often, these older citizens go to more than one physician and get medication for different problems from each doctor. The combination of the various chemicals can be deadly.

Furthermore, when doctors who treated Medicare patients were tested about their knowledge of prescribing medicine for these patients, a study revealed that 70 percent of them did not pass. Ironically, the majority of the M.D.s who were asked to be in the study refused to take the test at all. They said they had no interest in the subject of geriatrics and medication!

The drug companies are often guilty of inadequate testing. Nevertheless, they market the drugs to M.D.s, sometimes using skewed test results, misleading claims and slick advertising. The Food and Drug Administration (FDA) conducted a study in which it found that of 425 drugs commonly taken by older patients, only 212 had proper geriatric dosage and contraindication information supplied with them.

The risk of a bad reaction to drugs is thirty-three percent higher in those between fifty and fifty-nine than it is in people in their forties or younger. The FDA has reported that most of the deaths from prescribed drugs occurred in people who were sixty and over.

Below are statistics from the World Health Organization regarding a study on adverse reactions to drugs.

88% of all people had at least one problem with a prescribed drug.

22% of these patients have a possibly life-threatening condition perhaps caused by medication.

59% were given drugs that were either ineffective or contraindicated.

28% were given an incorrect high dosage.

48% were given drugs that had severe interaction effects when taken with other chemicals.

20% were given drugs that have the same effect of

other drugs they were already taking.

According to a 1993 report entitled, *Arthritis, Rheumatic Diseases, and Related Disorders*, published by The National Institutes of Health, more than 37 million Americans are afflicted by one or more of the rheumatic diseases. In addition, more than 25 million Americans have osteoporosis, and countless millions have other musculoskeletal disorders. The fact to remember is that drugs are not the first answer to physical problems. Drugs should be used as a last resort when all other natural methods fail.

"Chiropractic is the only science that exactly locates the cause of the dis-ease, then adjusts it."
— B.J. Palmer, D.C.

The drugs prescribed by medical doctors have serious side effects. For instance, aspirin may reduce pain and inflammation, but the sufferer may have to take eight or more tablets each day. This can cause stomach irritation, bleeding and ulcers. The non-steroidal anti-inflammatory drugs, such as Indocin, Advil and Naprosyn can cause kidney impairment, irritation and hemorrhage of the esophagus, stomach, duodenum and small intestine.

Doctors also prescribe steroids freely. Drugs like prednisone and hydrocortisone may offer some relief, but they make bones thin and weak. Gold Salts reduce inflammation, but they can create skin rashes and mouth ulcers.

"If you rush to take it (a new drug), do so with the full knowledge that you are being a guinea pig. The longer a drug is on the market, the more will be known about the side effects."
— Robert S. Mendelsohn, M.D.

NOTE: In April 1982, Eli Lily introduced Oraflex. It was removed from the market in August 1982 after seventy-three people died from the effects of the drug.

Medicine doesn't have an answer to the very real problem of osteoporosis, high blood pressure, menopause and other conditions associated with aging. For instance, menopausal women in their 40s and 50s, are given estrogen replacement therapy (ERT). By giving women small doses of the hormone estrogen, medical doctors have been able to slow bone loss but not renew bone mass. Furthermore, ERT can create serious long-term side effects, including an increased risk of breast cancer.

And other chemical therapy that's often prescribed to women is fluoride treatment. Not only is this non-effective; it also makes the bones more susceptible to fracture.

THE CHIROPRACTIC APPROACH

The fact is, the elderly need to be under the care of a chiropractor. When the chiropractor eliminates or reduces a patient's nerve interference, all the person's life support systems are strengthened and healing can occur naturally.

"There is no effect without a cause. Chiropractors adjust causes. Others treat effects."
— B.J. Palmer, D.C.

> **When 300 million people**
> **believe in a bad idea,**
> **it's *still* a bad idea.**

Chapter 9
A Dedication

To the late Robert S. Mendelsohn, M.D

Throughout this book, I have quoted from the works of a remarkable physician who is both an inspiration and a mentor to me. Robert S. Mendelsohn, M.D., was a physician but he became an outspoken detractor of the medical profession. In 1979, he published his best-selling book, *Confessions of a Medical Heretic*. He began it by saying: *I do not believe in modern medicine. I am a medical heretic. My aim in this book is to persuade you to become a heretic, too.*

Robert Mendelssohn raised a strong voice against the traditional hierarchy—and he knew what he was talking about. He was Director of Project Head Start's Medical Consultation Service and Chairman of the Medical Licensing Committee for the State of Illinois. He was honored numerous times with rewards for excellence in medicine and medical instruction. An advocate of a woman's right to have the best healthcare possible for herself and her child, he promoted home birth and spearheaded the grassroots' movement back to midwives who made house calls to help with the delivery.

In addition to *Confessions of a Medical Heretic*, he also wrote *Mal-e Practice . . . How Doctors Manipulate Women,* and *How to Raise a Healthy Child . . . In Spite of Your Doctor.*

He called hospitals *temples of doom,* and advised people to stay out of them at all costs, especially when a new baby was involved. In *Mal-e Practice* he said:

> *"An expectant mother should thank Providence for her good fortune if she has her baby in a taxi cab on the way to the hospital. The cabdriver may not be much help, but at least he will spare her from all of the purposeless, perilous, and unpleasant intervention her obstetrician had planned to inflict on her."*

He said that after a lifetime of working in them, he found hospitals to be the "dirtiest and most deadly places in town." He pointed out that every year approximately 1.5 million people contract infections in the hospital, prolonging their stay—but they are luckier than the 15,000 who die of the infection. He said doctors downplay this, calling the condition a *nosocomial infection* rather than the more accurate *hospital-acquired infection*.

Throughout his distinguished career, Dr. Mendelsohn was always ready to play David to modern medicine's Goliath.

As controversial as he was in the 1970s and 1980s, today, more and more of his theories are being validated. The movement towards fewer drugs, more natural healing and a naturally healthy lifestyle is a tribute to this man who is not afraid to speak out at a time when few we're ready to listen.

Since the beginning of my career, I have considered Robert Mendelsohn to be a real hero to all of us who have promoted natural healing first, before resorting to drugs or surgery.

It was sometime in the late 1970s, at a television talk show in St. Louis, Missouri, that I first met Dr. Mendelsohn. My wife and I were seated in the front row of the audience, and Dr. Mendelsohn was a guest along with a local radiologist. They had both been asked on the program to debate the many issues Dr. Mendelsohn discussed in his books.

This was at a time too, when I was just beginning to speak out on radio and television shows across the country. I knew instantly that I could learn a lot from this distinguished doctor who dared to forthrightly criticize the institution of modern medicine, of which he was, at the same time, an esteemed—and yet, an openly despised—member. I admired Dr. Mendelsohn, too, because he spoke for Americans who were the victims of chemical and surgical "overkill."

After the show, I expressed my gratitude to him for what he was doing. I saw the strength and courage he had to have to confront the *status quo* in his profession when he believed they were wrong. Dr. Mendelsohn's memory still inspires me as I try to follow his example in my own profession, praising the good and exposing the bad. And at those times when I am being ridiculed for doing so, I remember Dr. Robert Mendelsohn and smile.

Winifred Gardella's Experience

In the early 1950s Winifred Gardella it was a poster child for the March of Dimes. Her picture was published in the newspaper to raise huge sums of money for the March of Dimes in San Francisco. Nationally, her image raised millions of dollars to help fight the dreaded crippler, polio. Her sad, innocent face and her tiny body supported on crutches and leg braces, made many Americans reach into their pockets to donate.

But the March of Dimes couldn't help Winnifred. After two-and-a-half years under their doctor's expert care, her parents were told: "There is no hope."

Despite this dire prediction, her grandparents were determined to find a cure. They were not about to accept the opinion of so-called "medical experts." They decided to choose their own health care and they took Winifred to Dr. Lewis Robertson, a chiropractor. In less than six months of having her nerve interference corrected, Winnifred Gardella threw away her crutches and braces and went for a walk with her chiropractor. She has been walking ever since! (Search online: Winifred Gardella)

Chapter 10
Chiropractic Research

The chiropractic profession has always relied on clinical research and experimentation. In the 21st Century, chiropractic research is occurring around the world. Also, the chiropractic colleges are active in research, as are several excellent research organizations which adhere to the strictest scientific standards. This chapter presents a sampling of some of the most noteworthy research studies conducted since 1980.

- At Michigan's Oakland University, Miron Stano, Ph.D., compared the healthcare costs for medical and chiropractic patients. By reviewing the insurance claims paid, Dr. Stano concluded that patients who received chiropractic care, either alone or in conjunction with medical care, experienced healthcare costs that were $1000 lower on average than those who received only medical care. Total insurance payments for patients who received only medical care were 30 percent higher than those who were under the care of a chiropractor. This lower-cost was attributed to lower in-patient and out-patient costs and showed that "the chiropractic care substitutes for other forms of out-patient care."

- The Manga Report, from the University of Ottawa, reviewed all the international evidence on the management and low cost of back pain care. Pran Manga, Ph.D. concluded that significant cost savings would occur if the management of low back pain were transferred from physicians to chiropractors. He determined that chiropractic is safer than medical management of low back pain. "Many medical therapies are of questionable validity or are clearly inadequate. Chiropractic care is greatly superior to medical treatment in terms of scientific validity, safety, cost effectiveness and patient satisfaction." Dr. Manga concluded that "chiropractic should be fully insured (and) fully integrated into the Ontario health care system."

- The British Medical Research Council documented a ten-year study which compared chiropractic and hospital out-patient management of seventy-four patients with acute and chronic mechanical low back pain. The results showed that chiropractic care was significantly more effective than medical treatment for patients with chronic and severe pain. Furthermore, these results were long-term and remained consistent throughout the two-year follow up period. Chiropractic was also shown to save the British more than ten million pounds a year by having hospital out-patients with low back pain under chiropractic care.

- These findings reinforced the conclusions of the New Zealand report (377 pages) which was one of the most thorough and positive studies of chiropractic care on record. The twenty-month project was conducted by a government commission.

It concluded that spinal adjusting is a vital, very safe and clinically effective form of healthcare. Chiropractors have more thorough training in spinal mechanics and spinal care than any other health professional. Furthermore, chiropractic is scientifically-based and must be made an integral part of all hospital care. Finally, the report said that "modern chiropractic" is a soundly-based and valuable branch of healthcare in a specialized area neglected by the medical professional."

- J.S. Wright, D.C., conducted a study and reported to the *Journal of Chiropractic* that 74.6 percent of patients with recurring headaches, including migraines, were either cured or experienced reduced headache symptoms after receiving chiropractic adjustments. Daniel C. Cherkin, Ph.D. and Frederick A. MacCormack, Ph.D. administered a survey in 1989 that concluded that patients who were receiving care from health maintenance organizations (HMOs) in Washington State were three times as likely to report satisfaction with chiropractic care as they were from other physicians. The patient also reported they believed that their chiropractor was concerned about their welfare.

1992 Statistic:

Doctors in U.S.	Malpractice Premiums
Medical doctors	$ 41,971,000,000
Doctors of chiropractic	$ 62,500,000

- AV MED, A large HMO in the Southeast, wanted to see if it could save money by having patients visit chiropractors for back pain. They chose one hundred patients, eighty of whom had already been treated medically—without results. In each case, the patient had been seen by an average of 1.8 M.D.s. After receiving chiropractic adjustments, not one of the one hundred patients had to have surgery. Furthermore, eighty-six percent of them got better and none of them got worse. Herbert Davis, M.D., the medical director of AV MED, said that chiropractic care saved the HMO $250,000 in surgical costs alone!

- The State Industrial Insurance Systems (SIIS) in Nevada compared the average medical and chiropractic care for patients who suffered industrial injuries from 1988-1990. The results showed the 24.4 percent were back injuries but they accounted for more than 50 percent of all medical costs. Over the three-year period, the average medical cost per patient was $2142 which was 260 percent higher than the average chiropractic hospital cost per patient of $892.

Loss of work time under chiropractic care is less than one-third that for medical care. Furthermore, injured workers are able to continue working while receiving chiropractic care which may not be an option for medical care patients who are advised to have bed rest and medication. The Nevada Worker's Compensation Study emphasized that chiropractic eliminates the concern and expense of inappropriate hospitalization, unnecessary surgery, improper use of medication, including the high dosage of narcotic painkillers.

- In 1985, the University of Saskatchewan Study monitored 283 patients "who had not responded to previous conservative or operative treatment" and who were initially classified as totally disabled. The study revealed that after daily spinal adjustments were administered, "81 percent... became symptom-free or achieved a state of mild intermittent pain with no work restrictions."

- The *British Medical Journal* reported in the June 2, 1990 issue that T. W. Meade, M.D. studied patients over a two-year period. Dr. Meade found that "for patients with low-back pain in whom spinal adjustments are not contraindicated, chiropractic almost certainly confers worthwhile, long-term benefit in comparison with hospital outpatient management."

- In 1991, Steve Wolk, Ph.D., studied 10,652 worker's compensation cases in Florida. The results reported by the Foundation for Chiropractic Education and Research concluded that: "a claimant with a back-related injury, when initially cared for by a chiropractor versus a medical doctor, is less likely to become temporarily disabled, or if disabled, remains disabled for a shorter period of time; and claimants treated by medical doctors were hospitalized at a much higher rate than claimants cared for by chiropractors."

- The Gallup Organization conducted a demographic poll in 1991 which revealed that 90 percent of chiropractic patients felt their care was effective. More than 80 percent were satisfied with the care they received and almost 75 percent felt most of their expectations had been met during chiropractic visits.

- Also in 1981, Joanne Nyiendo, Ph.D., conducted a worker's compensation study in Oregon. She concluded that the median time loss in days for comparable injuries on any case was 9.0 days for patients who received chiropractic care as compared to 11.5 days for those who received medical treatment.

- Two years later, in 1993, researchers at the Royal University Hospital in Saskatchewan concluded that "the care of lumbar intervertebral disc herniation by side posture adjustments is both safe and effective." The researchers involved in the report, J. David Cassidy, D.C.; Haymo Thiel, D.C.; M.S. and W. Kirkaldy-Willis, M.D., are all on staff at the hospital's Back Pain Clinic.

- A 1992 review of data gathered from over two million users of chiropractic care in the United States appeared in the *Journal of American Health Policy*. It stated that "chiropractic users tend to have substantially lower total healthcare costs." The data also indicated that chiropractic care reduces the need for both physician and hospital care.

- *The Agency for Health Care Policy and Research (AHCPR) issues guidelines for low back problems.*

The U.S. agency for Health Care Policy and Research (AHCPR) formed a 23-person panel to find out the best ways to care for low back problems in adults. These healthcare professionals, including experts in orthopedic surgery, family practice, internal medicine, physical and rehabilitative medicine, emergency medicine, neurosurgery, rheumatology, and many other disciplines reviewed more than 3900 studies on the topic. These guidelines released in December 1994 verified what chiropractors had been saying for years: surgery and medication should be a last resort treatment for most cases. Moderate exercise and chiropractic adjustments are far more effective, and less risky.

Philip R. Lee, M.D. assistant secretary for health and director of the Public Health Service, said, "By encouraging people with acute low back problems to resume normal activities, using only those treatments that have been scientifically shown to be effective, these guidelines could save Americans considerable anguish, time and money now spent on unneeded or unproven medical care."

One clear message from all the studies is that chiropractic remains a cost-effective and efficient method of healing that is, in many instances, equal or superior to medical care. The studies, which have often been conducted by the state health or Worker's Compensation agencies, have shown that chiropractic is often less expensive, significantly reduces the time away from work and often eliminates the dangers of drugs and surgery.

According to a 1991 report by the Harvard Medical Practice Study Group in Cambridge, Massachusetts: 80,000 persons die every year—one person every 7 minutes— and 150,000 to 300,000 more are injured annually from medical negligence in hospitals.

A Measure of Malpractice, Harvard University Press 1993

By now you know health doesn't come in a bottle. However, the pharmaceutical companies want you to believe that reaching for their lotions, potions, powders and syrups will make you healthy. All it does is make them wealthy.

Chapter 11
Freedom of Choice

It's clear that when it comes to healthcare, the United States is anything but "the land of the free."

On every front, consumers and non-allopathic healthcare providers are struggling against a repressive and profit driven system which rivals George Orwell's worst "Big Brother" nightmare. Long ago the pharmaceutical and insurance industries formed an alliance with the medical establishment. Despite the court ordered truce that resulted from the Wilk case (see Chapter 12) these healthcare industries are continuing their push to discredit any methods or ideas which might loosen their stranglehold on the American public.

One report after another in the news media shows the medical, pharmaceutical,insurance monopoly targeting chiropractors. This establishment doesn't want doctors of chiropractic to threaten their complete control. Chiropractic currently represents only three-tenths of one percent of the total annual expenditure on healthcare in the United States.

As if they didn't have enough power, the medical community has also enlisted the help of an equally formidable opponent: the United States government. On every level—local, state and even federal—our rights to make personal and family healthcare decisions have been usurped. This violates our fundamental rights to "Life, liberty and the pursuit of happiness." Millions of Americans are lied to every year regarding medications. Encouraged by our government officials, the messages are enthusiastically broadcast by the local and national media.

NOT SMART ENOUGH?

If you should decide to choose treatment outside the organized and approved hierarchy of medicine, you will find it harder and harder to get insurance. You'll even get less compassion and understanding.

Stand at the border and watch the AIDS and cancer patients leaving for Mexico and Europe in hopes of finding treatment that doesn't exist in the states. We are denied access here to new medications and therapies, even when the condition has been diagnosed as terminal. Why? What's even more disturbing is medically aligned bureaucrats won't fully recognize chiropractic care, until we are shown to be scientifically validated. This sounds reasonable until you realize our government has hardly funded any research project for chiropractic when compared to medicine.

Unfortunately, many medical treatment guidelines

are devised by bureaucrats and claims adjuster's, and not by healthcare professionals. The over-riding consideration is financial instead of humanitarian. The pharmaceutical industry also adds to the problem. Physicians continue to prescribe drugs, because if they didn't the billion-dollar pharmaceutical industry would not survive.

Many are aware of this situation. It's a very real concern and an accurate assessment of the situation in America. Many chiropractors also believe our profession is often attacked by medicine and the media to divert the publics' attention away from the very real and well-documented dangers of drugs and surgery.

THERE'S NO "PROOF IN THE PUDDING"

"Only 15 percent of all medical procedures are scientifically validated."

— David Eddy, M.D., Ph.D.

Dr. David Eddy was the J. Alexander McMahon Professor of Health Policy and Management at Duke University in Raleigh-Durham, North Carolina. He received his M.D. degree from the University of Virginia, and a Ph.D. in engineering economic systems at Stanford University in Palo Alto, California. After serving on the faculty at Stanford as a professor of engineering in medicine, he went to Duke University in 1981 to set up the Center for Health Policy Research and Education. Dr. Eddy has developed policies for a number of organizations, including the American Cancer Society, the National Cancer Institute, the World Health Organization, the Congressional Office of Technology Assessment, the Blue Cross and Blue Shield Association and the American Medical Association. His mathematical model of cancer screening was awarded the Lanchester Prize, the top award in the field of operations research. Dr. Eddy serves on the Board of Mathematics of the National Academy Of Sciences and is a member of the Institute of Medicine.

When a man with Dr. Eddy's credentials claims that 85 percent of medical procedures have no scientific validation, it is important to the non-medical community to question the efficacy of modern medical practices.

M.D.s ONLY

Examine the directors serving in the healthcare agencies at any level of government. Most likely, you'll see a hierarchy that's completely dominated by M.D.s.

The question is: Who is making the critical decisions about our future healthcare? Average citizens, including

parents, doctors of chiropractic, or other alternative practitioners? No, the decision-makers are Johnson & Johnson,
Squibb, Merck, and all the other drug companies
supported by the insurance companies who resist paying
claims for anything outside the traditional medical venue.

SALES FIGURES FROM SECOND QUARTER, 1993

Company	Sales	Percentage increase over 1st quarter sales
Johnson & Johnson	$3 billion	+9%
Squibb (domestic)	$2.7 billion	+12%
Eli Lily	$1.4 billion	+12%
The Upjohn Co.	$859 million	+34%
Merck & Co.	$556 million	+12%
American Home Products	$265 million	+14%

These figures are for only three months April-May-June

In the first half of the 20th century many chiropractors went to jail for practicing their art. In spite of past
battles with organized medicine, our future is bright. Chiropractic is the largest non-medical healing system in the
entire world. This incredible "American discovery" is now

flourishing, but if we want natural health care to be available, we must be vigilant and protect our freedom of choice.

Dr. Harry Llewellyn's Experience

> "I was reading when I first felt a dull ache in my lower back. The ache continued on and off for days. I knew that a car accident in my childhood had caused a severe lordosis, or abnormal inward curvature of the lumbar vertebrae, but the injury had never affected me until now. Being a medical doctor, I followed the typical route of back x-rays and orthopedic surgeons. I was told I could avoid lying down on my back, tolerate the pain or try surgery. Not one of these answers appealed to me.

> "My brother-in-law advised me to visit a chiropractor. After a month of adjustments, I could read without any back pain. After five months of adjustments, I drove 18 hours back to New Jersey without any back pain. Until then my limit in a car was thirty minutes.

> "It's not the rapid recovery from pain that amazes me. It's my profession. As a medical

doctor, I had been an "alleged" non-believer in chiropractic. However, now I obviously believe in it. The pain in my right sacroiliac joint is gone. My knowledge of anatomy, physiology and biochemistry only strengthen my anticipation of the day when chiropractic is the brother of medicine."

Chapter 12
The Wilk V. AMA Case

It was a legal battle that continued for more than a decade. It was taken to the United States Supreme Court, and finally, a multi-million dollar Federal Appeals Court decision was rendered against the American Medical Association (AMA) and forever changed the course of healthcare in this country.

Nevertheless, a lot of people have never heard of *Wilk et Al vs. AMA*. Some might say this is because it lacked the drama of a Perry Mason court room or an episode of *L.A. Law*. Perhaps the antitrust issues were too complex for the general public to understand. There are some who claimed the powerful medical establishment suppressed the news. No one will ever know for sure.

THE VERDICT WAS "GUILTY!"

The guilty verdict in this case was an indictment of the AMA's lengthy attempt to illegally boycott the chiropractic profession.

The case began in 1976 when an Illinois chiropractor, Chester Wilk, and four other D.C.'s filed a restraint of trade complaint against the American Medical Association. At that time, the AMA labeled all chiropractors as "quacks" and went so far as to forbid its members from associating with them.

Working with investigators, the five chiropractors found evidence that the AMA's stand was motivated by economics. Chiropractors, along with other forms of alternative healthcare were becoming strong competitors in the healthcare marketplace. The AMA wanted to stop these "invaders" who threatened their turf.

A CAMPAIGN TO DESTROY

Throughout the years, as the case went through the courts, evidence mounted that the AMA had waged a systematic campaign to destroy the credibility of any alternative care health profession, particularly chiropractic. The worst part of this campaign was that people's health was affected—it was the patients who suffer the most.

On February 7, 1990, then US Court of Appeals judge Susan Getzendanner, upheld a District Court's decision which found the AMA guilty of conspiring with other medical healthcare organizations in a "lengthy, systematic, successful and unlawful boycott" designed to restrict co-operation between M.D.'s and chiropractors in order to eliminate the profession of chiropractic as a competitor in the United States Healthcare System.

The AMA appealed the case to the United States Supreme Court, but it was rejected. Judge Getzendanner's ruling stood.

The AMA complied with the court order and published the entire ruling in the *Journal of the American Medical Association (JAMA)* and the *American Medical News.* It also notified its members that they were free to refer to, accept referrals from, and associate with chiropractors.

M.D.'s & D.C.'s WORK TOGETHER

Long before the AMA lifted its band, medical doctors who were members of the association had begun to establish good business relationships with their chiropractic colleagues.

Judge Getzendanner rejected the AMA's "medical patient care" defense and cited scientific studies which proved that "chiropractic care was twice as effective as medical care in relieving many painful conditions of the neck and back, as well as related muscular and skeletal problems."

Since the courts findings and conclusions were released, an increasing number of medical doctors, hospitals and healthcare organizations in the United States have begun to include the services of chiropractors.

While it's going to take time for some diehards in

medicine to overcome their earlier negative indoctrination and personal prejudice about the "evils" of chiropractic—an alternate health care discipline—the Wilk case has opened the door for enhanced communication and cooperation between the two disciplines.

"We never know how far-reaching something we may think, say, or do today will affect the lives of millions tomorrow."
— B.J. Palmer, D.C.

Chapter 13
The Other Drug Problem

Because of its concern with the health of all people, the World Chiropractic Alliance (WCA) has become very active in the war on street drugs. The WCA is involved in community activities aimed at increasing public awareness about the dangers of illegal drugs, and engaged in a campaign to raise awareness of the legal drug problem worldwide. The legal drug problem is the misuse and abuse of prescription and over-the-counter (OTC) drugs.

While doctors of chiropractic recognize the value of some medications to relieve suffering or sustain life, doctors of chiropractic are almost unanimous in agreeing that, as a society, we take medications far too freely.

WORSE THAN COCAINE

Although it's seldom receives media attention, the *other drug problem* (prescription and OTC drugs) takes a larger toll, in terms of lives, health and money, than all the illegal hard drugs combined.

The current edition of the *Complete Drug Reference*

contains thousands of different medications. According to the FDA, there are hundreds of different OTC drug products available. Almost every one of these drugs, whether it's prescription or accessible over-the-counter, it can produce harmful side effects. Furthermore, many are highly addictive. One study showed that it's easier to get hooked on the commonly prescribed tranquilizer, Valium, than on cocaine or heroin.

HOW SAFE IS SAFE?

The truth is that even so-called "safe" drugs aren't totally harmless. In an average twelve-month period, more than 1.5 million hospitalized people suffer from the side effects of the drugs and therapy they receive there. Aspirin alone sends about sixteen hundred people to the hospital each year, of whom, die due to gastric bleeding.

Drug interaction also creates a serious problem. Some individual drugs may be relatively benign, but taken together, they can be deadly. According to the US Department of Health and Human Services, the average American senior citizen is given more than fifteen prescriptions each year. Sometimes, these come from doctors who aren't aware of the other medications the patient may be taking. This could lead to tragedy if the drugs cause a toxic reaction.

> **"All the drugs in the world cannot adjust subluxated vertebrae."**
> — B.J. Palmer, D.C.

WHO'S TO BLAME?

Why is the legal drug situation out of hand? We know that in the United States the medical doctors are part of the problem because they write one 1.6 billion drug prescriptions each year. In 75 percent of all office visits to an M.D., drugs are prescribed.

However, patients too, have to shoulder part of the blame. They seldom question their doctors and rarely request drug-free care, probably because most want a "quick fix" rather than a slower, more sensible approach to health.

Finally, a great deal of blame falls to the multi-billion dollar pharmaceutical industry which spends more than $10 billion each year to market its products, which is much more than they spend on researching the safety of taking these drugs.

It's clear the legal drug problem is driving the cost of healthcare up and the level of health down. Use of drugs also sends a dangerous message to our youth. Every time we put a pill in our mouths to calm stress, stop headaches, wake up or go to sleep, etc., we are telling our young people that "it's okay."

NOTE: if the tranquilizer, Prozac, is a reasonable alternative to dealing with problems, how much of a reach is it to use marijuana or cocaine—or worse?

Whether or not parents admit it, adults design the paradigms. It's the pattern we set that our kids follow. The next time you pop a pill, stop and consider what you're telling your children! It's up to you!

"Loss of life does not come from chiropractic adjustments: wish that we could say as much for surgical operations."
— B.J. Palmer, D.C.

The most dangerous part of receiving chiropractic care is driving your motor vehicle in traffic to the chiropractic office.

Chapter 14
Who Uses Chiropractic?

As stated before, Chiropractic is for everyone, not just blue-collar workers injured on the job, athletes with pulled muscles, accident survivors with whiplash, the very young or the elderly. Every year, more and more people of all ages and from all walks of life are turning to chiropractors to improve their performance. Ballerinas and quarterbacks... movie stars and politicians... golfers and singers... heavyweight champs and royalty are all among chiropractic's celebrity patients, past and present.

CHIROPRACTIC PATIENTS

BASEBALL: Ryne Sandberg, Brett Butler, Wes Parker, Don Sutton, Jeff Reardon, Roberto Clemente, Rick Monday.

BASKETBALL: Robert Parish, Jack Sikma.

BEACH VOLLEYBALL: Craig Moothart, Sinjin Smith, Kent Steffes, Tim Hovland, Randy Stoklos.

BODYBUILDERS: Arnold Schwarzenegger, Lori Ugolic, Franco Colombo, D.C.

BOXERS: Evander Holyfield, Jack Dempsey, Rocky Marciano, Tony Lopez, Michael Carbajol.

DANCERS: Marcelo Angelini, Daniela Buson.

ENDURANCE ATHLETES: Biathletes – Kenny Sousa, Joel Thompson, Brent Steiner and Fred Klevan. **Triathletes –** Mark Allen, Craig Reynolds, and Larry Rhoads.

ENTERTAINERS: Arnold Schwarzenegger, Shirley MacLaine, Mel Gibson, Meredith Baxter, Liza Minnelli, Bob Hope, Doris Day, Glen Campbell, the band Alabama, Roseanne Cash, Dixie Carter, Madonna, Cher, Linda Hamilton, Dennis Weaver, Richard Gere, Kim Bassinger, Alec Baldwin, will be Goldberg, Ted Danson, Macauley Culkin, Burt Reynolds.

FOOTBALL: Dammone Johnson, Alex Karras, Ricky Bell, Joe Montana, Mark Mays.

GOLFERS: Barbara Bunkowsky, Jan Stephenson, Amy Alcott, Donna White, Kim Bauer.

HOLLYWOOD STUNTMAN: Russell Towery.

OLYMPIC ATHLETES: Joseph Arvay (wrestling), Mary Lou Retton (gymnastics), Bruce Jenner (decathlon), Alberto Juantorena (400 & 800 meter run), Dwight Stones (high jump), Suzy Chaffee (skiing).

ROYALTY: Princess Diana of England.

RUGBY: Terrence Titus.

SKEET: Louise Kolar Terry.

SOCCER: Brian Haynes, Gregg Blasingame.

SURFER: Jeff Booth.

TENNIS: Tracy Austin, Jimmy Connors, Billie Jean King, John McEnroe, Ivan Lendl.

There are at least twenty-five million other people who are enjoying the benefits of regular chiropractic health care. If you are not one of them you need to ask yourself, why not? You cannot believe that you are doing everything for you and your family's health, if chiropractic care is not included in your life or your family's.

Please don't take your health for granted. Unfortunately, it is difficult for any individual to fully appreciate his or her health until it's gone, and when this happens the first symptoms may be the last one i.e. heart attack, stroke or kidney failure. Remember symptoms are the last thing to appear in a disease process.

And please, if you or your family members have not been screened for nerve interference—make an appointment today and make the effort to improve your health!

Chapter 15
The Chiropractic Principles

Chiropractic has many basic principles upon which all its philosophy, art and science is based. Those listed here are some of the most important. They have guided the profession since its earliest development. Some of them are almost universally accepted. Others are just beginning to find acceptance with other sciences. These principles follow a simple progression of deductive logic. If you accept the major premise, the other principles fall into place almost automatically.

THE MAJOR PREMISE

A Universal Intelligence is in all matter and continually gives to it all its properties and actions, thus maintaining it in existence.

THE SECONDARY PRINCIPLES

- The expression of this Intelligence through matter is the chiropractic meaning of life.

- Life is a Triune having three necessary unified factors, namely, Intelligence, Force and Matter.

- In order to have 100% Life, there must be 100% Intelligence, 100% Force, 100% Matter.

- A living thing has an Inborn Intelligence within its body, called Innate Intelligence.

- The mission of Innate Intelligence is to maintain the material of the body in active organization.

- There is 100% of Innate Intelligence in every living thing, the required amount, proportional to its organization. The amount of force created by Intelligence is always 100%.

- The function of Innate Intelligence is to adapt universal forces and matter for use in the body, so that all parts of the body will have coordinated action for mutual benefit.

- Innate Intelligence adapts forces and matter for the body, but is limited by the limitations of matter.

- The forces of Innate Intelligence will never injure or destroy the structures in which they work.

- The forces of Innate Intelligence operate through or over the nervous system in animal bodies.

- There can be interference with the transmission of Innate Forces.

- Interference with the transmission of Innate Forces causes dis-ease.

I AM A CHIROPRACTOR

I am a Chiropractor working with the sciences of the universe by turning on the life in man through the art of the adjustment. I do not prescribe, treat or diagnose conditions. I use only my hands. I work with that "mysterious something" which created my body from two cells.

At a time prescribed eons ago I was set in this body to experience. That cosmic power which created me, which also moves the seas, rotates the earth, directs the heavens, gives life, takes it away, is everything. And that power which set the universe in motion and created me did not abandon me when I became free of the security of my earthly mother's womb. It is still with me and protects me as it moves all forms toward their final predestined goal.

It is not mine to educatedly ask "why" or "where," but to Innately live; and live to help my fellow. And with this Chiropractic adjustment I use all the powers and energies moving this universe, to allow my fellow creatures the chance to live, free of dis-ease.

I wish nothing in return, only the chance to GIVE. I give with the only thing I have, LOVE. And I love all by removing that which interferes with 100% of LIFE. I do not look to others for direction, I look within. I am a perfect expression of God living 24 hours each day for others—I am a PRINCIPLED CHIROPRACTOR.

— B.J. Palmer, D.C., Ph.C.

THE BIG IDEA

A slip on the snowy sidewalk in winter is a small thing. It happens to millions.

A fall from a ladder in the summer is a small thing. It also happens to millions.

The slip or fall produces a subluxation. The subluxation is a small thing.

The subluxation produces pressure on a nerve. That pressure is a small thing.

That decreased flowing produces a dis-eased body and brain. That is a big thing to that man.

Multiply that sick man by 1000, and you control the physical and mental welfare of a city.

Multiply that man by 130 million, and you forecast and can prophecy the physical and mental status of a nation.

So the slip or fall, the subluxation, pressure, flow of mental images and dis-ease are big enough to control the thoughts and actions of a nation.

Now comes a man. And one man is a small thing.

This man gives an adjustment. The adjustment is a small thing.

The adjustment replaces the subluxation. That is a small thing.

The adjusted subluxation releases pressure upon nerves. That is a small thing.

The released pressure restores health to a man. This is a big thing to that man.

Multiply that well man by thousand, and you step up the physical and mental welfare of a city.

Multiply that well man by a million, and you increase the efficiency of a state.

Multiply that well man by a hundred thirty million, and you have produced a healthy, wealthy, and better race for posterity.

So, the adjustment of the subluxation to release pressure upon nerves, to restore mental impulse flow, to restore health, is big enough to rebuild the thoughts and actions of the world.

The idea that knows the cause, that can correct the cause of dis-ease, is one of the biggest ideas known. Without it, nations fall; with it, nations rise.

This idea is the biggest I know of.

— B.J. Palmer, 1944

B.J.'S LAST PRINTED WORDS

Time always has and always will perpetuate those methods which better serve mankind. Chiropractic is no exception to that rule. My illustrious father placed this trust in my keeping, to keep it pure and unsullied or defamed. I pass it on to you unstained, to protect as he would have you do. As he passed on, so will I. We admonish you to keep this principle and practice unadulterated and unmixed. Humanity needed then what he gave us. You need now what I give you. Out there in those great open spaces are multitudes seeking what you possess.

The burdens are heavy; responsibilities are many; obligations are providential; but the satisfaction of traveling the populated highways and byways, relieving suffering and adding millions of years to lives of millions of suffering people, will bring forth satisfaction and glories with greater blessings than you think. Time is of the essence.

May God flow from above-down His bounteous strengths, courage and understanding to carry on; and may your Innates receive and act on that free flow of Wisdom from above-down; inside-out . . . for you have in your possession a Sacred Trust. Guard it well.

GLOSSARY

ADJUSTMENT: The specific application of forces used to facilitate the body's correction of nerve interference.

ALLOPATHIC: Refers to conventional medicine as practiced by the graduate of a medical school which grants a medical degree.

ALVEOLI: Air cells of the lungs.

ANTIBODIES: Proteins manufactured by lymphocytes to neutralize foreign proteins, such as bacteria, viruses and other microorganisms in the body.

BASAL GANGLIA: Four masses of gray matter located deep within the brain.

CAPILLARIES: Small blood vessels.

CATATONIC: An unresponsive person refusing to move or talk, remaining in a fixed posture.

CEREBELLUM: A large portion of the brain connected to the brain stem and spinal cord. It coordinates voluntary muscular movements.

CEREBRUM: The largest portion of the brain consisting of two hemispheres. It receives information from the senses - sight, hearing, taste, and smell - through the brain stem and processes the data. It also deals with the higher mental faculties, such as thinking and comprehension.

CHIROPRACTIC: A primary healthcare profession in which professional responsibility and authority are focused on the anatomy of the spine and immediate articulation, and the condition of nerve interference. It is also a practice which encompasses educating, advising about and addressing nerve interference.

CHIROPRACTIC CARE LEVELS: There are three levels of care you will progress through when you are under the care of a doctor of chiropractic. The length of each care level is at the discretion of the practitioner and varies from patient to patient.

> **Level I Care:** A patient-specific number of visits, from daily to three times a week, with the objective of beginning the reduction of the clinical indicators of nerve interference. The duration of Level I Care is at the discretion of the practitioner.

> **Level II Care:** A patient-specific number of visits, from 1 to 2 times a week beginning with the first reduction of the clinical indicators of nerve interference with the objective of reducing clinical indi-

cators to a minimum level. The duration of Level II Care is at the discretion of the practitioner.

Level III Care: This is lifetime care with the frequency of office visits varying depending on the patient. It begins with the maximum reduction of the clinical indicators of nerve interference, and has the objective of sustaining the patient at that level.

CHIROPRACTIC DIAGNOSIS: A comprehensive process of evaluation of the spinal column and its immediate articulations to determine the presence of nerve interference and other conditions that may contraindicate chiropractic procedures. (See Medical Diagnosis.)

COMPENSATORY: To make up for or counterbalance.

DEDUCTIVE LOGIC: The Chiropractic Principle is based on this process of reasoning. A process of reasoning in which the conclusion follows necessarily from the major premise presented.

DIS-EASE: The word *disease* is a combination of *dis* and *ease*. *Dis* is a prefix meaning "apart from." It follows then the dis-ease is nothing more than a lack of comfort, a loss of harmony in the system. Chiropractors believe that instead of treating disease with chemicals and invasive procedures, whenever possible; first treat dis-ease with the reduction or elimination of nerve interference, thereby giving the patient a chance to recover naturally before resorting to drugs and surgery.

EOSINOPHIL: A type of cell of the peripheral blood or bone marrow whose granules stain red with eosin or other acid dyes.

EPIDERMIS: The outermost layer of skin.

ESTROGEN: Female sex hormones, estradiol and estrone, produced by the ovary. Responsible for the development of secondary sexual characteristics.

FIBRIN: A protein necessary for cells to form clots.

HEALTH: A state of optimal physical, mental and social well-being; not merely the absence of disease or infirmity.

HOMEOPATHY: A system of medicine, founded by Dr. Hahnemann in 1796 in Philadelphia, in which drugs are used in extremely small doses.

HOMEOSTASIS: The ability or tendency to maintain normal, internal stability and balance in an organism by coordinated responses of the organ systems. Examples of homeostatic mechanisms are the regulation of blood pressure, body temperature and blood sugar levels.

HYDROCHLORIC ACID: Normal constituent of gastric juice found in the stomach. Produced by the parietal cells of the gastric glands to serve many digestive functions.

HYPERACTIVE: Beyond or above normal behavior, excessive movements.

HYPERKINETIC: Excessive amounts of mobility. Similar to hypermobile.

LARYNX: The enlarged upper end of the trachea known as the organ of voice. It consists of nine cartilages bound together by elastic membrane moved by surrounding muscles.

LEUKOCYTE: A cell that acts as a scavenger and by so doing helps combat infection.

LETHARGY: A condition of sluggishness.

LIGAMENT: A band or sheet of connective tissue between the ends of bones that facilitate motion and support.

LYMPH NODES: A rounded body of lymphatic tissue of varying sizes that produce lymphocytes and monocytes. They act as filters to keep bacteria from entering the bloodstream. They also may stop cancer cells, but in turn may be the seat of cancer.

MANIPULATION: The forceful passive movement of a joint beyond its active limit of motion. It doesn't imply the use of precision, specificity or the correction of nerve interference. Therefore, it is not synonymous with chiropractic adjustment.

MARROW: Tissue inside the long bones of the body. Red marrow is involved with the production of blood cells.

MAST CELLS: Cells which are present in most body tissues but most prevalent in connective tissue, such as the innermost layer of the skin. They play an important role in the body's allergic response because they release chemicals responsible for allergic symptoms into the tissue.

MEDICAL DIAGNOSIS: Procedures that provide information about disease processes for the selection of treatment.

MEDULA OBLONGATA: The lower portion of the brain stem and the enlarged part of the spinal cord in the skull.

MELANIN: The pigment which gives color to hair and skin, etc.

METABOLISM: The rate and sum of all the physical and chemical changes that take place within the body.

MRI: *Magnetic Resonance Imaging* or MRI uses a combination of radio waves, magnetic fields, and computers to create a high-quality picture of the internal organs, the soft tissue and the nerve network. Like the CAT Scan, the patient lies motionless while being passed through a narrow cylinder. It can detect brain and spinal tumors, disc disease, spinal stenosis, degeneration and indications of a stroke. It's also used to examine heart and liver tissue and the joints. This is the method that is preferred for examination of spinal disc degeneration.

MYELOGRAPHY: The Myelogram procedure includes a "spinal tap" which is used to get information on spinal cord compression and disc problems. A needle is inserted between the lumbar vertebrae, spinal fluid is drained and replaced with dye, and then the patient is X-rayed. There are risks inherent in this procedure. Some patients may develop severe headaches that can last for several weeks or months. Others are allergic to the dye which can stay in the body for years. Furthermore, the results are not entirely accurate. Myelography is being replaced by MRI and CAT Scans.

NERVE INTERFERENCE: See vertebral subluxation.

NEUTROPHILS: A leukocyte which can be readily stained by neutral dyes.

NOSOCOMIAL INFECTION: An infection contracted as a result of being hospitalized.

OSTEOPATHY: Originally, a system of medicine based upon the theory that the normal body is able to rectify itself against toxic conditions. While some manipulation is still used to treat patients, most osteopaths today rely heavily on drugs and surgery to treat patients.

OSTEOPOROSIS: Increased porous condition of bones with bones becoming soft.

PAPILLAE: A small, nipple like protuberance or elevation.

PARKINSONS: A chronic nerve disease characterized by a fine, slowly spreading tremor; muscular weakness and rigidity.

PARASPINAL EMG SCANNING: A painless, non-invasive procedure to measure and record the electrical signals given off by the muscles that attach to the spinal column. Electrodes are placed on the skin and their readings are shown in the form of a graph. Since one of the symptoms of nerve interference is abnormal muscle activity, the EMG is becoming a popular method for charting most muscle spasms and spinal imbalance.

PEPSIN: The chief enzyme of gastric juice which converts proteins.

PHALANGES: The bones of a finger or toe.

PYLORUS: The lower opening of the stomach into the small intestines.

RENNIN: A coagulating enzyme found in the stomach of cud-chewing animals which curdles milk.

TARSAL BONES: The seven bones of the ankle.

THERMOGRAPHY: This procedure measures the temperature on the skin surface to locate inflammation of muscles and soft tissues. A special camera takes pictures which reflect the different temperatures by displaying a range of colors on film. Thermography has been used to pinpoint spinal nerve and muscle stress.

TRIUNE OF LIFE: The name for the three elements which influence every living organism: Innate Intelligence, Innate Energy and Innate Matter.

VERTEBRAL SUBLUXATION: Also referred to as nerve interference, is a misalignment of one or more of the 24 vertebrae in the spinal column, which causes alteration of nerve function and interference to the transmission of mental impulses, resulting in a lessening of the body's Innate ability to express its maximum health potential.

VESTIGIAL: A bodily part or organ that is small and degenerate or imperfectly developed in an earlier stage of the individual.

VITALISM: The doctrine that teaches that in living organisms, life is caused and sustained by a vital principle distinct from all physical and chemical forces. It also teaches that life is, at least in part, self-determining and self-evolving.

X-RAY: The common name for *Radiograph* which is a picture of the solid parts of the body produced by passing electromagnetic rays through the body positioned against photographic film. The rays pass through the soft tissues but are stopped by metal and other solid objects, like the bones including teeth. The X-ray tube was invented by Wilhelm Roentgen in 1895, the same year D.D. Palmer discovered chiropractic. His son, B.J. Palmer, established one of the finest X-ray laboratories in the country because he realized the contribution X-ray diagnosis would make to spinal analysis.

REFERENCES AND FOOTNOTES

I've intentionally not listed references or footnotes throughout the text. I wanted to avoid interfering with the concentration of the reader. Anyone interested enough to research the contents of this book will find the list of references to be more than adequate source material. These references are offered for suggested reading material as well as confirming the validity of the statements and contents of this book.

HISTORY OF CHIROPRACTIC

Dye, A. August: *The Evolution of Chiropractic: It's Discovery and Development*. Richmond Hall, Richmond Hill, NY 1969.

Maynard, Joseph E: *Healing Hands: the Official Biography of the Palmer Family.* Fourth Edition. Jonorm Publishers, Woodstock, GA 1991.

Moore, J. Stewart: *Chiropractic in America: the History of a Medical Alternative.* Johns Hopkins University Press, Baltimore, MD 1993.

CHIROPRACTIC PHILOSOPHY

Bach, Marcus: *The Chiropractic Story*. DeVorss & Co. Los Angeles, CA 1968 reprinted by Si-Nel, Marietta, GA.

Barge, Fred H.: *Life Without Fear.* Barge Chiropractic Clinic, LaCrosse, WI.

Dintenfass, Julius: *Chiropractic: A Modern Way to Health,* Pyramid Books, NY 1975.

Koren, Tedd: *Bringing Out the Best in You.* Koren Publications, Philadelphia, PA 1994.

Koren, Tedd: *World's Greatest Drugstore.* Koren Publications, Philadelphia, PA 1977 and 1994.

Rutherford, Leonard W.: *The Role of Chiropractic.* Clinton Press, Inc., Erie, PA 1989.

Strauss, Joseph: *Your Amazing Body.* Lifeline Publications, Levitown, PA.

HEALTH AND HEALING

Chopra, Deepak: *Quantum Healing.* Bantam Books, New York, NY 1989.

Moyers, Bill: *Healing and the Mind.* Doubleday, New York, NY 1993.

Siegle, Bernie: *Love, Medicine and Miracles.*

INSIGHTS ON TRADITIONAL MEDICINE

Carter, James P.: *Racketeering in Medicine.* Hampton Roads Publishing Company, Norfolk, VA 1993.

Inlander, Charles B., Leven, Lowell S., Weiner Ed: *Medicine on Trial.* Pantheon Books, New York, NY 1988.

Mendelsohn, Robert S.: *Confessions of a Medical Heretic.* Contemporary Books, Chicago, IL 1979.

Mendelsohn, Robert S.: *Malepractice.* Contemporary Books, Chicago, IL 1982.

Mendelsohn, Robert S.: *How to Raise a Healthy Child in Spite of Your Doctor.* Ballantine Books, New York, NY 1984.

Schmidt, Michael A., Smith, Lendon H., Sehnert, Keith W.: *Beyond Antibiotics.* North Atlantic Books, Berkeley, CA 1993.

Speransky, A.D.: *A Basis for the Theory of Medicine.* Translated and edited by C.P. Dutt. New York International Publishers 334, 1943.

Szasz, Thomas: *The Theology of Medicine.* Syracuse University Press, Syracuse, NY 1988.

Wolfe, Sidney M.: *Worst Pills Best Pills.* Public Citizen Health Research Group, Washington, DC 1988.

CHILDREN AND CHIROPRACTIC

Biedermann H.: Kinematic Imbalances Due to Suboccipital Strain In Newborns. *Manual Medicine* 6(5):151, 1992.

Briegel, Louis R., Stefanski, Stacey A.: *For the Love of Children.* Innate Publishing, Canton, GA 1993.

Blessing S.J.: What You Should Know About Ritalin. *Chiropractic Pediatrics* 1(1):16, April 1994.

Collins K.F., Barker C, Brantley J. et al: The Efficacy Of Upper Cervical Chiropractic Care On Children And Adults With Cerebral Palsy: A Preliminary Report. *Chiropractic Pediatrics* 1(1):13, April 1994.

Golden L., Van Egmond C.: Longitudinal Clinical Case Study: Multi-disciplinary Care Of Child With Multiple Functional And Developmental Disorders. *J Manipulative Physiol Ther* 17(4):279, 1994.

Goodman, R., Mosby J.: Cessation Of A Seizure Disorder: Correction Of The Atlas Subluxation Complex. *Journal of Chiropractic Research and Clinical Investigation* 6(2):26, Feb 1991.

Gutmann G.: Blocked Atlantal nerve Syndrome In Infants And Small Children. English translation in *International Review of Chiropractic* 46(4):37, July 1990 Original German paper published in *Manuelle Medizin* 25:5, 1987.

Klougart N., Nilsson N., Jacobsen J.: Infantile Colic Treated By Chiropractors: a prospective study of 316 cases. *J Manipulative Physio Ther* 12:281, 1989.

Koren Tedd: Muscular Dystrophy and Chiropractic: The Eric Knapp Story. *Chiropractic Pediatrics* 1(1):18, April 1994.

Langley C.: Epileptic Seizures, Nocturnal Enuresis, ADD. *Chiropractic Pediatrics* 1(1):22, April 1994.

Marko R.: *Bed Wettings: Two Case Studies. Chiropractic Pediatrics* 1(1):21, April 1994.

Masarsky C., Weber M.: Somatic Dyspnea And The Ortho-
pedics Of Respiration. *Chiropractic Technique* 3(1):26, Feb
1991.

Phillips N.: Vertebral Subluxation And Otitis Media: a case
study. *Journal of Chiropractic Research and Clinical Investigation* 8(2):38, July 1992.

Rubinstein H.: Case Study: Autism. *Chiropractic Pediatrics*
1(1):23, April 1994.

Schimp J., Schimp D.: the Neuropathophysiology Of Trau-
matic Hemiparesis and Its Association With Dysfunctional
Upper Cervical Motion Units: a case report. *Chiropractic
Technique* 4(3):104, Aug 1992.

Schutte B., Teese H., Jamison J.: Chiropractic Adjustments
and Esophoria: a retrospective study and theoretical dis-
cussion. *J Manipulative Physiol Ther* 12:281, 1989.

Van Breda W., Van Breda J.: A Comparitive Study Of The
Health Status Of Children Raised Under The Health Care.
Journal of Chiropractic Research 101, Summer 1989.

Woo C.: Post-traumatic Myelopathy Following Flopping
High Jump: a pilot case of spinal manipulation. *J Manipulative Physiol Ther* 16(5):336, 1993.

IATROGENIC (DOCTOR CAUSED) ILLNESS

Bedell, S.E., Deitz, D.C., Leeman, D., Delbanco, T.L.: Incidence and Characteristics of Preventable Iatrogenic Cardiac Arrests. *JAMA* 265(21):2815, June 5, 1991.

Begley, Sharon: the End Of Antibiotics. *Newsweek,* March 28, 1994.

Dye, Michael: Silent Danger Of Medical Malpractice: third leading cause of preventable death in U.S. *Public Citizen* May/June 1994. Public Citizen Health Research Group, Washington, DC.

Evans, R.S., Classen, D.C., Stevens, L.E., Pestotnik, S.L., etc. al.: Using a hospital information system to assess the effects adverse drug events. *Proc Annu Symp Comput Appl Med Care:* 161, 193.

Ferner, R.E., Whittington R.M.: Coroner's cases of death due to errors in prescribing or giving medicines or to adverse drug reactions: Birmingham 1986-1991. *J.R. Soc Med* 87(3):145, Mar 1994.

Stremple, J.F., Bross, D.S., Davis, C.L., McDonald G.O.: Comparison of Postoperative Mortality and Morbidity in VA and Nonfederal Hospitals. *J Surg Res* 56(5):405, May 1994.

Quires Torres, G., Hernandez, J., Reyes, A.: Iatrogenic Diseases in Surgery of the Ear. *Rev Laryngol Otol Rhinol (Bord)* 114(1):25, 1993.

Robin, E., McCauley, R.: The Malpractice Crisis and the Rate of Actual Malpractice. *Adm Radiol* 13(1):20, Jan 1994.

Stambouly, J.J., Pollack, M.M.: Iatrogenic Illness in Pediatric Critical Care. *Crit Care Med* 18(11):1248, Nov 1990

Steel K., Gertman P.M., Crescenzi C., Anderson, J.: Iatrogenic illness on a general medical service at a university hospital. *New England Journal of Medicine* 304(11):638, Mar 12, 1981.

About the Author

Dr. Terry Rondberg is a prominent leader in the chiropractic profession. He started private practice in 1975 after graduating from Logan College of chiropractic. Over the next fifteen years he helped thousands of patients in his offices in St. Louis, Missouri and Phoenix, Arizona.

Reaching thousands wasn't enough for Dr. Rondberg. He knew that throughout the country, around the world, there were millions of others who had not yet experienced the power of chiropractic firsthand. Sadly, he also knew that there were millions more who probably never would have that opportunity. They were either cut off from chiropractic care because of unfair insurance practices or they were led to believe that conventional medical treatment was the only avenue to health.

These are the people Dr. Rondberg wanted to reach through an intensive campaign of public education and political action. In 1986, he founded *The Chiropractic Journal*, a monthly newspaper distributed to every chiropractor and chiropractic student in the world. He uses the pages of his phenomenally successful publication to help build a stronger profession and safeguard it from its detractors.

In the years since he has published *The Chiropractic Journal*, he has seen the chiropractic profession achieve many of its goals, including a victory in the Wilk vs. AMA lawsuit, and recognition by numerous government agencies.

In 1989, he widened his horizon even more and founded The World Chiropractic Alliance, a non-profit "watchdog" organization dedicated to promoting a vertebral subluxation-free world. Time and again, the organization has led the fight to protect the consumers' right to choose chiropractic as their first choice in healthcare. With massive public relations efforts, he has won chiropractic support from people around the world, and has helped inform millions of individuals about the philosophy, art and science of chiropractic.

Reflecting both the depth of his knowledge and the enthusiasm of his convictions, Dr. Rondberg has become a popular speaker at chiropractic conferences, conventions and seminars. A prolific writer, he has also authored numerous publications and articles on chiropractic for both the profession and the public.

Dr. Terry Rondberg's latest book, *Bioenergy Breakthrough: Nourish Your Brain, Restore Your Health,* released in 2015, is available in paperback, Kindle and audio book, through online and retail bookstores.

To learn more, visit: www.bioenergycertification.com

WORLD CHIROPRACTIC ALLIANCE

Are chiropractic and its drug-free approach to healthcare an important issue for you? Have you found relief, avoided surgery or discovered how your family can benefit from regular visits to your chiropractor to maintain wellness and build natural immunity?

Do you feel the government or insurance companies have the right to choose the type of healthcare you should have access to?

Even though chiropractic is the world's largest natural healing profession, unfair managed care programs, legislators and insurance companies are quickly closing the door on your freedom of choice regarding healthcare. This is clearly an organized effort to once again eliminate chiropractic as a healthcare choice for consumers.

The World Chiropractic Alliance (WCA) is a nonprofit organization made up of chiropractors and chiropractic consumers. The purpose of the WCA is "Promoting a Vertebral Subluxation Free World."

The WCA is a watchdog organization ready to challenge any group or organization that threatens the chiropractic practice objective. The WCA will fight any discrimination against chiropractic consumers. We need your help to protect your constitutional rights—your fundamental right to choose your mode of healthcare.

Join us.

Contact and questions:
www.worldchiropracticalliance.org